Praise for
Hello, Higher Self

"Bunny's exploration of conversations with the Higher Self have been so enlightening for me since I started following them on socials years ago. This book is the perfect compilation of these explorations and an expansion on the beautiful concept/truth of our Higher Selves. Leaning into their love and vision for us can be a catalyst for transformational healing of the wounds left from our traumas in this reality."

— Singer and LGBTQ+ rights activist Lauren Jauregui

"*Hello, Higher Self* achieves the elusive balance of motivating us to work toward everything that we deserve without ignoring the material conditions of the world that we're experiencing. This book is a powerful read full of tools—some revolutionary, some practical—that help us to tap into the power that we already possess."

— Michell C. Clark, author of *Eyes on the Road*

"Bunny Michael gives me hope for the future. *Hello, Higher Self* is a vulnerable and inspirational manifesto for creative misfits and sensitive souls, reminding us that authenticity is more important than perfection, all true love begins with self-love, and the wisdom of the Higher Self is just one shift in perception away. If you've ever felt like an outsider, or excluded by traditional definitions of spirituality and success, welcome home. This book is for you."

— James McCrae, author of *The Art of You*

"*Hello, Higher Self* is the book I wish I'd had my whole life. Bunny opens up a whole new world—one in which we can all too clearly see the ways in which we have been conditioned to hate, fear, and shame ourselves and each other. Knowing that they can't leave us here, Bunny offers roadmaps for how we can move back toward love, compassion, and care—toward creating the kind of world that we've always deserved. *Hello, Higher Self* is a gift to us all."

— Writer and educator Margeaux Feldman of @softcoretrauma

Hello, Higher Self

An Outsider's Guide to <u>Loving Yourself</u> in a <u>Tough</u> World

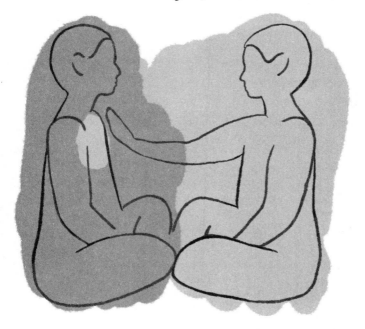

Bunny Michael

VORACIOUS

Little, Brown and Company

New York   Boston   London

Copyright © 2024 by Bunny Michael

Hachette Book Group supports the right to free expression and the value of copyright. The purpose of copyright is to encourage writers and artists to produce the creative works that enrich our culture.

The scanning, uploading, and distribution of this book without permission is a theft of the author's intellectual property. If you would like permission to use material from the book (other than for review purposes), please contact permissions@hbgusa.com. Thank you for your support of the author's rights.

Voracious / Little, Brown and Company
Hachette Book Group
1290 Avenue of the Americas, New York, NY 10104
voraciousbooks.com

First Edition: June 2024

Voracious is an imprint of Little, Brown and Company, a division of Hachette Book Group, Inc. The Voracious name and logo are trademarks of Hachette Book Group, Inc.

The publisher is not responsible for websites (or their content) that are not owned by the publisher.

The Hachette Speakers Bureau provides a wide range of authors for speaking events. To find out more, go to hachettespeakersbureau.com or call (866) 376-6591.

Little, Brown and Company books may be purchased in bulk for business, educational, or promotional use. For information, please contact your local bookseller or the Hachette Book Group Special Markets Department at special.markets@hbgusa.com.

Print book interior design by Bart Dawson
Illustrations by Bunny Michael

ISBN 9780316471565
LCCN 2023951112

Printing 1, 2024

MRQ

Printed in Canada

Dedicated to everyone I call family.

(You know who you are.)

May we continue to grow from

each other's mistakes and triumphs.

Contents

Preface

You Are Enough

Every day you log on to your phone and are confronted with an existential crisis. The twenty-four-hour news cycle tells you about another mass shooting, a dire statistic on climate change, the death toll of international conflicts, and another case of police brutality. You log on to your social media accounts to check the stats on your digital identity to see how you measure up compared to your peers. Your avatar is on display around the clock, vulnerable to any criticism—especially self-criticism.

Your morning ritual is supposed to set you up for another day of striving for success, status, and acceptance, but instead it just reminds you how broken the world is: the inequality, the injustice, the need for social change. Like a virtual mirror, it shows you what you like about yourself, and what you don't. What people like about you, and what they don't.

And all before breakfast.

No wonder so many of us feel overwhelmed. No wonder it's difficult to feel hopeful about the world. No wonder the journey to healing can feel so long and hard—or even sometimes impossible.

Which is where *Hello, Higher Self* comes in. This book provides revolutionary and practical tools for staying connected to your "Higher Self" daily: my term for the part of us that knows, no matter what, that *we are enough*.

The truth is everyone feels like an outsider trying to fit into an image of what success, beauty, social status, health, and spirituality look like. Because the world has taught all of us that we must prove we belong.

I have built an audience of hundreds of thousands of followers with this Higher Self message. Along the way, I have received thousands of comments and messages from followers telling me how much they needed this content. Very often I get a comment that says, "How did you know I needed this today?" And my response is almost always the same: "Because I needed it too. We are on the same journey."

Most of all I have seen the emotional and mental fallout from an entire generation roaming the internet without guidance, leadership, or protection, and I've witnessed the ways in which online activity directly (and often negatively) impacts people's lives offline. A life lived online is new to so many of us, and people are scared, feeling isolated, and desperate to find their truth. Connecting to your Higher Self means finding your own source of truth and power and remembering your innate worth in a world of biased beauty standards and egomaniacal pursuits of status.

The time has come for all of us to channel our power. This is a guidebook for an inner awakening that will transform your outer reality. Every time you choose to see yourself through the lens of your Higher Self, you help shift the collective consciousness from pain and oppression to peace and equanimity.

Loving yourself changes the world. That's how important you are.

Hello, Higher Self

When you were born, you had a natural inclination to love yourself just as you are. You allowed yourself to be cared for without ever questioning whether you deserved it.

But then you got older, became socialized, and were taught that in order to be "good enough" you needed to look a certain way, accomplish certain things, and have certain possessions. Feeling the pressure to prove your worth began in your childhood: Am I smart enough? Am I good-looking? Does my family have a nice car? Am I too fat? Too skinny? Is my skin too dark? Am I good at sports? Do people like me?

Your parents, caregivers, and teachers instilled these beliefs by mirroring what was taught to them as children. Popular culture—movies, TV shows, and advertisements—gave you visual cues of what beauty and success were supposed to look like. When you didn't look like the characters on TV, or you weren't the smartest kid in class, or you experienced neglect and abuse, you wondered what was wrong with you.

Feeling like an outsider, you internalized what you saw was lacking in your life as a signal that you yourself were lacking.

You are not alone.

Growing up queer in a conservative Mexican and Samoan family in Texas forced me to find my inner voice. It forced me to find my own source of love and follow my Higher Self guidance. I've felt like an outsider my whole life because I didn't fit the image of what my parents wanted. I struggled as an artist because I didn't have the confidence. I looked for a spiritual teacher for guidance, but no one seemed to be addressing the issues that I wanted answers to, such as how to deal with being queer and nonbinary and living in a racist and sexist world. Connecting to my Higher Self meant finding my own truth, knowing my worth, unlearning limiting beliefs and biases to experience my wholeness. When I started listening to the voice inside me that said *You've always been enough just how you are,* everything changed. I realized trying to fit in only made me smaller. Following the path of my Higher Self expanded all possibilities.

Our entire adult lives, we're made to feel that if only we had more, did more, or changed in some way, we would be better than who we are now, and we could climb higher up the social hierarchy to reach the promise of happiness, acceptance, and fulfillment.

This formula for self-worth is an illusion, and always has been.

In truth, your success, money, status, productivity, or possessions do not equal your value.

You have been deceived. We all have.

We never had to prove we are worthy of love, care, safety, and abundance — we are worthy, simply by being ourselves.

Your Higher Self is who you are beyond your hierarchical conditioning; the wisdom of the love that you were born with, the knowledge that you are already whole. In order to access the power of your Higher Self, you must bring to light the unconscious beliefs that have imprisoned you in the illusion of your inadequacy.

My term for the conditioning by which we have grown so accustomed to judging ourselves against the world around us is **Learned Hierarchical Beliefs (LHBs).** LHBs have been passed down from generation to generation as a way of organizing society along the lines of status, wealth, and power. The foundation of LHBs is that your value depends on where you are on the hierarchy of human worth.

Race, class, gender, sexuality, social status, and body image are just some of the measurements that determine your value as a person, according to LHBs. This fundamental principle—the idea that some people are worthier than others, or more deserving of love, success, or abundance—is why there is so much unnecessary human suffering in the world, and why you have struggled with self-worth and personal fulfillment.

Accessing your Higher Self is the process of unlearning your LHBs, corresponding to a 180-degree shift in your perspective and your reality, from "I am not enough" to **"I am enough and always have been."**

At the heart of human suffering is a deep fear of unworthiness. Left unchecked, a culture dominated by LHBs is a culture of greed, inequality, and conflict, both internal and external. Choosing the path of your Higher Self is a radical shift to prioritize unlearning, self-care, and compassion for other people. It's understanding that every human is in a different stage of unlearning these hierarchical beliefs, and in a different stage of healing the trauma that resulted from growing up in a culture dominated by them.

Your LHBs may be the loudest voices in your head, trying to convince you to see the world through a lens of lack, scarcity, and unworthiness. But with practice, and using the tools I will give you in this book, not only will you begin to debunk the false belief that you are not enough, but your life will become more joyful and fulfilling. And the biggest bonus? If we all work together to recognize LHBs for what they are and reject them by embracing our Higher Selves, we will transform the world.

Harnessing the power of your Higher Self can be broken down into five steps.

1. **Become witness to your thoughts.** Most of the time you are not consciously aware of what you are thinking. You are just reacting to your thoughts unconsciously. The first step to subverting the influence of your LHBs is to begin to notice them. For example, what are you telling yourself in a

moment when you are feeling insecure or unhappy about how you look? What beliefs do you have about your own self-worth around your career or relationships? You are not your thoughts; you are the awareness behind your thinking. We will go over practices in this book that will help you hone this step.

2. **Investigate where those thoughts come from.** Most people accept that their childhood experiences influence how they see themselves. We can spend hours unearthing those experiences in talk therapy, but fail to realize that so much of the pain we go through personally is rooted in a collective belief system that does not value us. Most of us are undereducated about the historical context of our cultural biases and how they perpetuate trauma, because most of our education has been whitewashed and sugarcoated.

   We have all been raised in a racist, patriarchal, ableist, homophobic, transphobic, fatphobic, and classist world. No one is immune to that conditioning. LHBs feed cycles of abuse, neglect, and suffering, because in a system of dominance, there is no room for healing and compassion. In a system of greed, there is only scarcity.

   When you learn about where these beliefs come from and why you are influenced by them, it becomes much easier to separate who you really are from what your LHBs tell you. That is why this book spends extensive time on the historical context that influences our cultural bias today.

3. **Replace your negative thoughts with the voice of your Higher Self.** Treating yourself with love and compassion may seem like a challenge. Even though it is your nature to love yourself, it can feel unnatural if you are not used to it. Your Higher Self is communicating to you all the time, but as with a radio broadcast, if you are not on the right station, you will miss the message. Choosing to hear the voice of your Higher Self takes intention and practice.

Once you have built an awareness of the thoughts you want to change and expanded your understanding of why those thoughts are there in the first place, you can replace them with loving ones that will empower you. There are many ways to channel your inner voice of love, because we all come from different experiences, backgrounds, and relationships to language and ritual. In this book I cover a variety of methods: free writing exercises, visualization, meditation, rituals, and journal prompts. Experiment with these modalities to find what works for you. You can also use your creativity and intuition to develop your own methods of accessing your inner wisdom. There is no right or wrong way.

4. **Change your behavior to support your relationship to your Higher Self.** When you start accessing the voice of your Higher Self, you will notice the patterns of behavior in your life that make it more difficult to follow your Higher Self's guidance. We need to recognize those patterns and then subvert them. Sometimes it can be as small as reducing the time you spend on your phone or spending more time with friends who are on a similar path. I will give you a road map to help you hear the voice of your Higher Self more clearly and more often.

5. **Never stop repeating steps 1, 2, 3, and 4.** No matter how much awareness, unlearning, and practice you have under your belt, you live in a world that is unpredictable and chaotic, and is set up to profit from you continuing to buy into LHBs. No matter how much your understanding of your relationships has changed, you can still get triggered, and your feelings can still be hurt. This isn't a quick fix. This is not a master class where you walk away "fixed." There is no finish line when it comes to awakening to love and your Higher Self. This is an ongoing process of evolving your consciousness. There are no limits to the possibilities of where that evolution can take you. It's challenging, but it's also extremely freeing and rewarding.

How to Use This Book

Each of the following eighteen chapters focuses on a different area of life, such as dating, gender, body image, sex, social media, race, and politics. Each chapter will provide clear steps to becoming aware of how you have been socially and culturally conditioned to approach this area from an "I am not enough" perspective, before illustrating a Higher Self perspective, helping you transform that part of your life with the confidence that you are enough.

Each chapter will also include a personal story showing how I discovered my Higher Self, because while our paths might look different, our journey is the same.

Although topics are separated by chapters, many are interconnected. For example, while body image and racism are interwoven, I highlight them individually to help clarify how to address each one. Furthermore, when it comes to cultural and historical Learned Hierarchical Beliefs, this book could not possibly cover everything. Each chapter could be its own book. My attempt here is to crack open the veneer—to take you on an expedition in the underground cave of our collective disillusionment with one flashlight. Every surface will not be uncovered, but you will begin to see the layers—and, I hope, keep exploring on your own.

One last thing before you get started: This book isn't about providing you with the right way to live your life. This book is intended to connect you to the part of yourself that knows what is right for you. You are wise, creative, and a gift to this world. You have always been lovable. You have always been enough. It's time to step into your power.

I am so honored to be on this journey with you.

All my love,

Bunny

Chapter 1

Social Media

> **Me:** *Why am I so anxious about what other people think about me?*
>
> **Higher Self**: *The validation you have been seeking outside yourself is creating anxiety because you are looking where you can't find it. In truth, it's been inside you the whole time.*

Chasing Likes

One beautiful Sunday morning, my first thought upon waking was *I need to check Instagram.* I felt around for my phone, tapped on the app, and got that familiar feeling in the pit of my stomach: the dread of finding out how many likes yesterday's post got. *Was it a success?* I checked the stats. Nope. It didn't perform well. The number of likes was below my average. A couple of nice comments but nothing extraordinary.

The anxiety in my stomach turned to a sinking feeling. I felt hurt and rejected. *What am I doing wrong?* I reexamined my post. It was my most recent self-portrait: a digital collage in a high-definition virtual paradise with palm trees and pastels — like

Frida Kahlo meets Disneyland. It took me hours to make it in Photoshop. The night before, I really liked it. I had fun making it. I felt like it was a moment of growth as an artist. But the following morning, all I felt was embarrassment. *Why was I so stupid to think this was good?*

Then I scrolled through my profile and analyzed the few posts that *had* received a lot of likes. *What did I do here that I didn't do last night? Is it the colors? Is it the way my body looks? Is it my hair? Is it the stupid look on my face?* I was a detective holding a magnifying glass to every detail of my post, hoping to catch the flaw that had precipitated my failure. When I didn't get an answer, I scrolled to look at other people's posts, still investigating. I took note of whose posts were getting more likes than me and why.

They are better-looking.

They are more talented.

They have a larger following.

My work is so much better than theirs. I don't get why people like them so much.

They are famous. I wonder if I'll ever be famous.

If only I had what they had, my life would be so much better.

I spent the better part of 2016 in this perpetual state of social media hell. I wanted so badly to win the war of personal achievement, and Instagram had become my battleground. Unlike Facebook, where only people who were already successful outside the platform had huge Facebook followings, people were actually becoming successful *through* Instagram. From the moment I moved to the city, my attempt at becoming a professional artist in New York was a roller coaster of successes and failures. I believed that Instagram could be the answer to all my prayers—if I was good enough to make it happen.

My desire to be successful on social media was all about attainment of status. But wanting the approval of as many people as possible didn't begin with the invention of Instagram or Facebook or any other app. That message was received many years earlier.

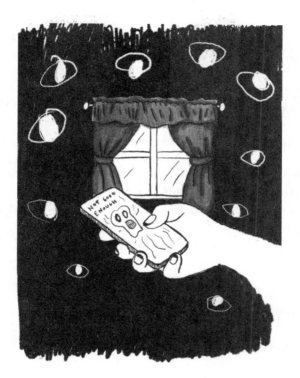

Learning to Fit In

At a young age we were taught self-worth is determined by how well we win the approval of caregivers, educators, and our peers. Standardized grade systems trained us to quantify our intelligence by how high or low we score compared to other students. Random adults commented on and compared our appearance — from body size to texture of hair. We compared our looks to the characters from movies and TV shows that perpetuated mostly Eurocentric and fatphobic beauty ideals.

For most of us, our behavior growing up was put into two categories: that of a "good girl" or "good boy," which meant following the rules, listening to authority without question, and being able to sit still and pay attention. Being a "bad girl" or "bad boy," on the other hand, meant not listening, not following directions, and acting out in school. It didn't matter what your home life was like or how confusing and arbitrary the rules were. It didn't matter if the educational system was terribly outdated and valued only certain types of learners and test-takers. The pressure was on us to fit into the mold, to be "good," and the more approval we gained in socialized environments, we were led to believe, the more we could value ourselves.

We were kids who were made to feel we had to please the adults around us, perform better than our peers, and raise our social status to be accepted. So we did our best to do just that. But our self-worth was never dependent on how we looked, behaved, or performed in school. We have always been inherently worthy.

I wanted to be popular.

One day in the fourth grade my teacher, Ms. Turner, told our class to divide into groups of our choosing and come up with something to make and sell at our school fundraiser. My friend Lauren waved to me from her seat on the other side of the room and flashed me a huge smile indicating she wanted to be in a group with me. I smiled back and gave a thumbs-up. Lauren was a little shy like me and always wore pastel dresses, with her strawberry-blond hair tightly pulled back by a thick plastic headband accentuating her big rosy cheeks. At recess, we asked another girl to be in our group, and decided we'd make lanyard bracelets.

Then after school, Marissa approached me. She and her two best friends (Jennifer and Jennifer) were the most popular girls at school. Marissa had mousy brown hair and bright green eyes and always talked about soccer practice and Indian Princesses (the appropriative wilderness program where mostly white men and their daughters wear headdresses and go camping). Her mom drove a shiny new minivan, was never late picking her up, and packed Marissa the best snacks, like Fruit by the Foot or Ritz mini crackers with cheese. In shock, I quickly let go of my little sister's hand and took one backpack strap off my shoulder because only losers wore straps on both shoulders.

"Hi, me and Jennifer and Jennifer wanted to know if you want to join our group for the fundraiser. We are making friendship bracelets!" Marissa asked.

Is this really happening?

"Yes!" I said.

"Oh cool, we can plan more with the group tomorrow in class." And in a flash, Marissa disappeared behind the sliding maroon door of her mom's Chrysler Town and Country.

The next day at school I avoided Lauren. I didn't know how to tell her we weren't going to make lanyard bracelets together. When Ms. Turner told us to get up and join our groups after lunch, I just went over and sat next to Marissa. The look on Lauren's face was of total confusion and disbelief. I was only ten years old, but I knew being in a group with Marissa and the two Jennifers was a step up for me. I didn't particularly like them—in fact, one of the Jennifers was really annoying. But being their friend meant popularity, it meant status, it meant there was something good about me. It meant I was better than Lauren.

From that day on, being popular became a priority. If I had to ditch less "desirable" friends, even if they were nice and accepting of me, so be it. I didn't want the bad feelings that came with not being good enough for the popular girls. I wanted to be cool, admired, and envied. It was proof that I belonged. If the popular kids liked me, that meant everyone else did too. I was already chasing likes.

Comparing Yourself to the Entire Internet

Social hierarchies have always existed, but like so many other aspects of our lives, technology transformed those hierarchies from analog to digital, expanding not only the amount of time we spend in a day thinking about our social standing in relation to others, but also exponentially multiplying the pool of people we now compare ourselves to in just a matter of a few minutes of scrolling.

It's . . . a lot.

The genius of social media is that it gives us the ability to quantify social hierarchies. Like the number in our bank accounts, our social worth is tallied in a currency of followers and likes. And just as many people believe the more money you have, the happier you are — in the digital world, the more social clout you have, the more you "matter." So why wouldn't you strive to build up your followers and likes? Why wouldn't you feel like something was wrong with you if you have less?

A lot of people tell me they often feel ashamed of themselves for being jealous or always comparing themselves to others on social media. But isn't that what you were trained to do — to judge how well you are doing based on your spot on the hierarchical ladder? You can't be a winner if there aren't any losers.

Trying to be good enough is exhausting.

Not long after my disappointing Disneyland-meets-Kahlo IG post, I clocked out of an excruciating brunch shift, during which a customer let their three-year-old pour an entire bottle of ketchup all over the table without helping to clean it up, and walked to my local bodega to grab a bag of Utz chips, a grape kombucha, and a pack of Little Debbie powdered donuts. When I got to my apartment, I headed straight to my room to avoid running into my roommate (I had used the last of his coffee that morning), and got into my bed — an Ikea mattress on the floor. Then I began my daily ritual of scrolling on Instagram. Everywhere I looked it seemed like everyone was doing so well: becoming successful with their art, in a loving relationship, having fun with a huge group of friends. Fear and anxiety started building up inside me.

I'm so pathetic, I thought. *Here I am in my thirties with no partner, still waiting tables, and no foreseeable success. I'm failing at everything.* Memories flashed before me: the time I thought I was getting a record deal but it fell through, the time I got kicked out of my college's fine arts program, the way my mom looked at me when she asked how my career was going, my ex's face when she said she wanted me to move out.

Instagram was bringing all of it to the surface.

Everyone could see how poorly my posts were doing, and my ex was seeing someone new. On social media it felt like my life was on stage, my flaws were under the spotlight, and the audience was my family, my peers, people I was both inspired by and jealous of, and strangers who might visit my page but not find me interesting enough to follow. I had hoped social media would make people see me the way I wanted to see myself — successful, cool, popular, and talented. But I was failing at that, too. *I hate myself,* I thought. I started to cry.

My tears made my liquid eyeliner drip into my eyes, and they started to sting. *Dammit.* I went to the mirror in the bathroom to wipe my face, and gazed at my reflection. "I'm such a mess," I said out loud. Then, to my surprise, I laughed a little. It was pretty comical: the makeup on my cheeks, the white powder from the donuts I ate earlier at the corners of my mouth, me standing there talking to myself in the mirror. I started to calm down, started to breathe deeper and slower. *You're okay.* As I lay back down in my bed, I thought about what I'd just said. *You're okay. Who's okay? If I'm okay, then who is telling me that I'm okay? Is that me, too?*

"I'm tired of trying to be enough," I said out loud. And then my own voice answered me back internally: *So stop trying. You already are enough and you always have been.*

Hearing that voice was disorienting, yet somehow it felt totally familiar, like in a dream when you know you are in your house but it looks nothing like your house. "Stop trying" to be good enough? I had never thought about it that way.

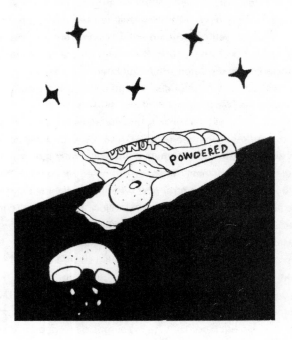

Up to that point in my life it seemed like self-loathing was going to break me, but when I heard that voice, a light began to shine through the cracks from somewhere deep within my consciousness. *You are already enough,* it said. *You always have been.*

Why is it so hard for me to believe that about myself? I thought. Then I remembered the trauma I've been through:

how my parents didn't accept me being gay at a young age, the racism I experienced growing up, the abusive relationship I had survived. For the first time, I was looking at myself with a deep sense of compassion. *You deserve better than the way you have been treating yourself.*

I was terrified that there was something fundamentally wrong with me, and my relationship to social media—this place where it is so easy to compare myself to others and put myself down—exacerbated the problem, I realized. The likes are there for a reason. To rate myself. To accumulate validation. To show that some people are better than others. How could I have felt like I was enough when I was putting my worth in the hands of a piece of technology I couldn't control?

The deepest level of my being sensed that this inner voice was telling me the truth. I didn't need to change. My perspective did. I didn't have a name for the voice, the feeling, the kind of love that spoke to me from my heart with total compassion and acceptance. But as I lay in my bed—on mascara-stained sheets sprinkled with donut crumbs—I experienced a profound shift. I couldn't see my worth because I was looking for it in the wrong place. My worth lay *within* me, not *outside* me. I needed to learn to love and accept myself.

I kept crying—no longer with tears of sadness, but with a profound sense of letting go.

No Amount of Likes Will Make You Like Yourself

The reach of social media has both enforced social hierarchy and highlighted its empty promise of personal fulfillment. Take a look around online and you will see people with all the supposed social "status" struggling to find that unapologetic self-love they were born with. Celebrities and influencers are becoming more candid about the pressures of fame and its impact on their mental health.

People with political power and influence are behaving like insecure teenagers and picking petty fights on X (formerly known as Twitter). Internet trolls, fearing their own inadequacy, spend countless lonely hours at their computers DM-ing, stalking, and harassing the mostly female, queer, or trans people they claim to be better than.

Why? Because **when you equate who you are with where you rank in a made-up hierarchy, one self-imposed by your Learned Hierarchical Beliefs, you will wake up one morning with a profound feeling of emptiness.** It's not just the people who are lower on the social hierarchy that suffer—it's everyone. When you do not know how to value yourself, no amount of outside validation is enough. When you don't know how to value yourself, you will not be able to see the inherent value in others. You will suffer and you will cause suffering.

Who we are on social media is a curated image, an attempt to control the way we are seen by others. But no matter the filters, the captions, or the selfie angles, we can't control anyone's judgments and opinions of us. **What we see in other people online is a projection of how we see ourselves.** If you are choosing to be online—or are required to by your job or to connect with communities that matter to you—bringing your Higher Self with you can greatly reduce the suffering that can come from time spent in an environment that can so toxically reinforce LHBs.

Remember Who You Really Are

Your Higher Self has always been inside you. Who you really are doesn't go away just because you are not conscious of it. The more mindful you are of what your thoughts tell you while you are online, the more you will see that *you have a choice whether or not to believe them.* The process of unearthing your LHBs about social media is just a matter of paying attention to the narratives that go through your mind when you are on or thinking about social media, and getting curious and contemplating where your beliefs and assumptions are stemming from. Where does your fear of not being good enough come from? Who is speaking when you say to yourself that you are failing because you don't have thousands of followers?

Your Higher Self is the compassionate awareness behind your thinking, not judging you or putting you down for your self-loathing thoughts or bouts of jealousy (only LHBs would put you down!) but reminding you with love that there is a new way of looking at this, one indicative of how worthy you always have been. You can come out of the darkness of illusion and step into the light of your truth. Aligning with your Higher Self is a practice, and it's not easy, but neither is the constant up and down of chasing that outside validation.

You are not your LHBs. You are your Higher Self, and your Higher Self is calling bullshit on all of this.

In order for my perspective to change, I had to make different choices.

In the days that followed my initial experience of hearing my internal voice of self-acceptance, I became more conscious of the moments when I was putting myself down. I also began to see patterns in my behavior online that were making me more vulnerable to self-loathing thoughts. So, I made some changes. I blocked my ex's profile so I couldn't see her posts, I unfollowed people who triggered negative feelings about myself, and if I noticed I was starting to feel bad, I logged off Instagram and did something else. These changes made a difference in my state of mind, but I sensed there was still more I could do.

Then one day a friend of mine DM-ed me with a popular meme. It was a picture of two different Kermit the Frogs facing each other in conversation, but one of the Kermits was wearing a black cloak reminiscent of a Star Wars Sith Lord. Each version of the meme was a variation of an internal dialogue between regular Kermit and evil Kermit, who represents the "negative" perspective. For example, one version:

Me: *I'm going to be more social, go out with friends, and enjoy life.*
Also Me: *Alienate all your friends because they secretly hate you.*

Another version:

Me: *He's always been sweet and trustworthy.*
Also Me: *Suspicious. Break into his phone and look through his texts.*

Self-deprecating meme culture was taking off, and even though I found it funny and entertaining, I thought, *Wow, this is not what I need right now. I don't want to reinforce my negative self-image—I want to see myself differently.* Then I had an idea. What if I make my *own* version of that meme, but instead of Kermit, I do a photo collage of two of me? I could write from a higher perspective, the voice inside me that reminds me of how worthy I really am. I took two selfies—one looking upset, and the other calm, loving, and patient—and I collaged them together. I wanted to create the meme version of the experience I had that day in the mirror. It was in this moment that I finally came up with a name for my inner voice. In proper meme language I wrote on the top of the image: **When Your Higher Self Tells You to Face Your Shit.**

I didn't know if the meme was good or if people would like it, but I didn't care. It came from an experience that had shifted my perspective for the better. I posted it. I felt deep satisfaction finally expressing my true experience, not a projection of what I thought other people would want. It felt healing. Then I realized that if I was going to continue to channel my Higher Self perspective—the acceptance that I am enough—I needed to do more than change my habits online. To continue to exist on this higher plane, I needed to intentionally seek that perspective within my own consciousness. It was too easy to slip back into my low self-image—there was too much pressure to fit in. I needed to hold myself accountable.

I decided that every day I would dedicate time to looking within myself and bringing that inner voice of love into my conscious awareness. And I would use Instagram as a platform to share that voice. Basically, I was subverting everything my Learned Hierarchical Beliefs intended me to feel—all of the unworthiness, competition, and pain got flipped on its head. By *me*.

From Micro to Macro: We All Need Our Higher Selves

My method for creating the memes consisted of bringing self-loathing and limiting thoughts into my awareness, understanding the reasons I had become stuck in those thought patterns, and then replacing the automatic thought with one from the perspective of love and compassion.

Two things I understood very quickly:

1. It wasn't difficult to notice the mean things I said to myself because I said them all the time.
2. Understanding my personal experiences didn't go far enough to root out the cause of my limiting beliefs. I needed a deeper understanding of the societal structures that produced those experiences.

It wasn't enough to know that my parents were homophobic at the time I came out as a teenager—I wanted to bring more awareness to the conditioning that led them to that perspective. It wasn't enough to just say my abusive ex was a jerk—I was interested in understanding how toxic masculinity perpetuates abuse.

It finally clicked for me. **The Higher Self perspective meant seeing the world through a new lens** with which you are able to separate the human from their conditioned beliefs. People struggle with self-worth because for generations we have been inundated with cultural messaging and trauma that have convinced us we aren't good enough. Those beliefs are passed down. The people who had hurt me were caught up in the same desperate illusion of needing to be better than other people; like me, they were ignorant of their inherent value. Outwardly, the effects of their false beliefs might have manifested differently than mine, but inwardly, the perspective was the same. Everywhere I turned, I saw these hierarchies playing out. Social media was just one medium for expressing them. I understood that the Higher Self perspective wasn't just about helping myself—it was about tearing down the whole system.

Watch Out for Sneaky LHBs

In many ways social media platforms have helped popular culture outgrow some of the racist, sexist, ableist, homophobic, and transphobic LHBs that we grew up with. Now anyone who has access to the internet has visibility, a voice, and a potential audience. There's an influx of body positivity, gender- and sexuality-affirming communities, and progress around decolonizing beauty standards.

Social media has helped educate and inform the masses regarding important issues around politics, race, gender, and class. But LHBs are sneaky and can change shape. Like a snake that sheds its skin only to reveal its new suit, Learned Hierarchical Beliefs can evolve with the culture. There are hierarchies within activist movements; there's judgment within spiritual communities. If you're not mindful, someone who is just like you, sharing their authentic self on social media, can become your competition rather than who they should be—a potential friend. Hate groups use social media to manipulate and indoctrinate young people, and misinformation can spread like wildfire. It's hard to determine if social media as a whole is healing or hurting us as a society. But there is no stopping it—the further into the future we go, the more time we are spending online.

Social media can also be a blessing when it comes to unlearning your LHBs, because it can bring more awareness to the ways in which you judge yourself and other people. But unless you take that further step of realizing that climbing up the ladder of social clout does not actually fill the void of your own self-worth, you will forever be stuck in the cycle of needing more and more external validation. No amount of followers and likes will ever be enough to make you feel like you are enough. You will forever be focusing on what you don't have, that one negative comment, or that person who unfollowed you (whom you don't even interact with anyway). When you are stuck in the mental framework of your LHBs, the entire game is about climbing higher and higher. Only, you will never reach the top because the top is an illusion. Seeing the world through the lens of your Higher Self is a total dismantling of this hierarchical system, no matter what guise that system takes.

No one is better than anyone else. Period.

It's a Practice, Not a Goal

Five years and over a thousand Higher Self memes later, I'd love to tell you that I never get caught up in self-limiting thoughts on social media. But that's not how it works. Just a few weeks before writing this, I caught myself in another downward spiral brought on by fears of inadequacy. My posts get thousands of likes now, but if I don't stay mindful of where my thoughts are taking me, five thousand likes might as well be negative five thousand. Because when I let my LHBs take over, all I can see is lack. It's never been about the number. And it never will be. The only way to feel like you are enough is to acknowledge that you always have been.

Learned Hierarchical Beliefs are very difficult to let go of. It takes self-compassion, practice, and patience. So below are some guidelines, affirmations, and journal prompts to help you on your journey.

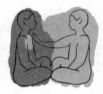

Bring Your Higher Self with You Online

1. **Know why you are logging on:** Instead of mindlessly opening Instagram, TikTok, or any other app just because your phone is nearby, ask yourself, *Why do I want to look at this now? Is it to compare myself to other people or to be inspired? Is it to find a way to feel better about myself by judging other people? Or is it to connect with other people? Or am I just bored?* Getting clear on why you're logging on gives you more control over your experience. If you can't find a good reason to log on, don't.

2. **Give yourself time limits:** Your Higher Self knows that your mental and emotional health is your number one priority. No amount of social media success, even if it helps your career, can replace your inner well-being. Even if you have to post every day for your job, you don't have to also scroll for three hours a day. Set reasonable goals by starting with small changes. Become aware of how many hours a day you are on the apps. Start with taking one hour off a week until you are on for a max of only one hour a day per app. One hour a day is plenty of time to post and catch up with what you have missed. Make sure to take at least one day off a week.

3. **Check in before you type anything:** When you post something online, it is permanent—even if you delete it, there could be a screenshot documenting it. Think about how many times you have said something you regret IRL. Online, there is no apology that will be sufficient to everyone. Before you type anything, ask yourself, *Who is speaking now? Is it my Higher Self, or is it my LHBs trying to make someone feel small so I can feel better about myself? Is this something I want someone to hold me accountable for five years from now?* If you're still not sure if you should say it—don't. There will be plenty of opportunities to voice your truth when you are clear on your intentions.

4. **Being called out on social media can be a gift:** The term "cancel culture" has been so misused by both progressives and conservatives that it has lost its meaning. Truthfully, no one who is being held accountable online for their behavior changes unless they want to, which requires an inner shift in awareness of how their LHBs have potentially caused harm. Yes, there are people who simply want to bully others to feel empowered, but in my experience, most of the call-outs on social media are acts of love—people who are speaking out on behalf of generations of marginalized people who did not and do not have a voice; people who want a more compassionate and just world; and people who, through their own emotional labor, are filling the void of lack of education around our hierarchical system that has left so many behind. If your behavior is being questioned online, ask your Higher Self, *What can I learn here?* before you react defensively. It doesn't mean that every online criticism is justified, but it does pose an opportunity to grow, if you are willing to look within.

5. **Unfollow, block, restrict, mute:** Social media is not a safe space. There are people who go online with the intention of causing harm. They are human just like you, but that doesn't mean you have to put up with any form of their abuse. Thankfully, many social media apps have tools to help protect you

from harassment, although nothing is foolproof. Use every tool at your disposal. Your Higher Self knows that any person who feels the need to be hateful and abusive online is acting from their own wounds and in need of healing. When you remind yourself of this, it helps to lessen their power to hurt you. It isn't about you. It's as if they are speaking to themselves indirectly. Engaging with abusers online, even if it's to defend yourself, makes you vulnerable to more abuse.

6. **Think of social media as an opportunity to make a positive impact rather than a challenge to gain social clout.** When we think about making a positive impact, we often think we must save the world; but often, a positive impact is simply sharing love with your family and friends. Being an example of compassion, authenticity, and self-acceptance, no matter how large or small your online community is, makes a tremendous impact on our collective consciousness. Brightening someone's day by making a funny TikTok can be so healing. Having the courage to share your art on social media can inspire someone else to have the courage to share theirs. Sharing your feelings can help someone feel less alone. At its essence, social media is a form of communication. So what is it that you want to communicate? What really matters to you?

7. **Most people on social media aren't judging you — they are too busy judging themselves. (And if they are judging you, it's because they are indirectly judging themselves.)** When you are stuck in your LHBs, it's difficult to see outside that system. It's a filter that prevents you from seeing the truth, which is that we are all searching for the same thing — love and acceptance. But we all go about it in different ways. From the perspective of your LHBs, you need to be better than other people in order to be lovable and accepted, and that is why it's so easy to find yourself online, judging other people and yourself. From the perspective of your Higher Self, love is within

you, and the acceptance that you have been searching for is self-acceptance.

LHBs About Social Media vs. Your Higher Self

LHB: The more likes and followers you have on social media, the more valuable you are as a person.

Higher Self: Social media apps are run by private companies that use algorithms to "predict" user preferences and tailor user experiences. They do this to keep users on the app for as long as possible, so they can gather data to sell to other companies. Content that is likely to get the most negative emotional response gets the most engagement. So no matter how authentic you are as a person on social media, the statistics of likes and followers will never be an authentic representation of you. It is what the algorithm determines as valuable, aka how monetarily valuable you are to the company.

LHB: People with more influence on social media have happier lives.

Higher Self: If your happiness is dependent on your influence on social media, you are letting your happiness be determined by circumstances you cannot control. In truth, real happiness comes from total self-acceptance of who you are right in this moment. Regardless of social status. Often people with a lot of influence on social media have to learn this truth the hard way.

LHB: You shouldn't show your flaws on social media.

Higher Self: The more you accept yourself, the more authentic you will be wherever you show up—in person or online. The more authentic you are, the more you encourage and inspire authenticity in your community of friends and peers. This is how you help transform the world from the limits of Learned

Hierarchical Beliefs to the joy and equanimity of a society that reflects our Higher Selves.

LHB: Who people are on social media is an accurate representation of their true selves.

Higher Self: Who people are on social media is a projection of where they are in their journeys of healing and self-acceptance. Everyone is in a different stage of that journey. The way people behave online most often has nothing to do with you. So don't assume you know what is going on in someone's life by how they present themselves on social media.

LHB: I will always be insecure online.

Higher Self: You're basing your security on what other people think about you, which is really a reflection of how they feel about themselves. How can you be secure about something you can't control? When you focus on treating yourself with kindness, compassion, and care while engaging online, you will feel grounded in the security of your indisputable self-worth.

Journal Prompts

1. When I am on social media, I mostly feel...

   _____

2. The things I don't like about social media are...

   _____

3. My biggest insecurity on social media is...

   _____

4. Some personal experiences that contribute to my insecurity on social media are . . .

_____

5. The social and cultural beliefs that affect how I see myself on social media are . . .

_____

6. Some ways that I judge people on social media are . . .

_____

7. Flip the script: What would my Higher Self say about my value on social media . . .

_____

8. Some changes I can make to my social media habits to embrace my Higher Self online are . . .

_____

9. When I log on to social media, my Higher Self wants me to remember . . .

_____

10. I can share love on social media by . . .

_____

Chapter 2

Creativity

Me: *I really want to be more creative, but I'm afraid I'm not good enough.*
Higher Self: *Creativity is self-expression. How can you not be good at expressing who you are? There is no other you.*

I've always been a weirdo.

From the earliest I can remember, people told me I was weird. As a young child, my favorite thing to do was talk in a gibberish language I'd invented that sounded like an alien version of Dora the Explorer speaking in tongues. I'd put on little performances where I'd contort my body and make distorted facial expressions that were more like theater of the absurd than the typical six-year-old playing pretend. "You are so weird!" my sisters and cousins would say, as they cracked up laughing, watching me run in circles making strange noises, my arms flapping like those inflatable figures outside car dealerships.

I didn't feel weird. I was just being myself, and these characters I'd embody mirrored the abstract nature of my imagination—they were explorations in shapes, colors, and textures. My oddball improvisations made people laugh, and I relished the attention. Being called weird made me feel special. My parents saw this behavior as me being a quirky, imaginative child. There was nothing wrong with it—until there was.

"If you keep making those ugly faces, one day your face is going to stay like that." My mom's words sent a jolt to my tiny ears like the unexpected shock I'd get grabbing a fresh T-shirt out of the dryer. She was clearly not entertained by the freakish smile I was making at myself in the passenger mirror, riding home from the grocery store. I was pretending to be a woman I'd seen on TV, leading a church congregation with mystical blue eyeshadow and overdone mascara. I didn't realize my mom was watching.

My mom is beautiful and took pride in how my sisters and I looked. Her Samoan upbringing taught that no matter where you are, you are representing your family. My strange quirks and ridiculous faces were okay up to a certain age, but that day in the car, I was almost eight and it no longer looked cute to her.

With her comment echoing in my mind, I felt like the boy Adam I'd read about in *Bible Stories for Young Children*. I had been frolicking in a garden of my own imagination, and then was told I was naked, that I should be embarrassed. I realized being "weird" wasn't special. It was ugly, and my mom was worried I might become *permanently* weird.

Stifling Creativity

When we were children, we were encouraged to creatively express ourselves: finger painting, crafts, drawings, music, dress-up, and make-believe. Teachers, parents, and caregivers would ooh and ahh over a bunch of scribbled lines. "Great job!" they'd say when we'd sing a song. They'd hang our stick figures on the refrigerator and encourage us to hokey pokey with abandon. Watching us express ourselves creatively provided a window for our caregivers to understand our thoughts and feelings.

But the older we got, the less we were encouraged to be creative for our own self-expression. Creativity became like everything else in school—there was a hierarchy of good and bad. We all experienced a turning point where the definition of "artistic" began to mean *someone who possessed a certain talent*. If your diorama didn't receive as much praise as your classmate's, or you couldn't sing an A when your music teacher tapped on that triangle, you suddenly weren't *good* at drawing or you weren't *good* at singing. Many of us were discouraged from creativity because it didn't fit into what was socially acceptable. Boys were discouraged from taking ballet, teenagers who wore black lipstick and dyed their hair were treated like troublemakers, schools in marginalized neighborhoods lacked funding for the arts because Black and Brown kids were not expected to grow up to be classical musicians. Being an artist meant fitting into predetermined criteria, and if you didn't meet those criteria, what would be the point of continuing to explore your creativity?

The Myth of Good and Bad Art

Most people would say that art is subjective. But throughout history, some people's subjective opinions on what is *good* or *bad* art have mattered more than others. For generations, a very small group of people have decided who were the so-called geniuses of their craft. These were the artists who not only were technically adept, but did work that conveyed a message meaningful to the dominant culture; what that artist had to say became important.

There is no such thing as good or bad art. There is only what is meaningful, inspiring, and relatable to you. In Western civilization, the artists who have received the most recognition have been white cis men who were speaking to the tastes and relating to the artistic perspectives of other white cis men (even if they were borrowing from other cultures without giving credit).

Art is self-expression. The reason our culture isn't aware of the inherent value of everyone's self-expression is because in a system based on a hierarchy of human worth, some people's self-expression is assigned more value than others'. We see examples in art history that clearly show how the hierarchical lens through which art is seen directly influences its cultural value.

Pablo Picasso's travels to Africa and encounters with the work of Indigenous artists there directly influenced some of his most renowned work, without Picasso ever crediting his sources. Paul Gauguin's portraits of nude Tahitian women and girls (some as young as thirteen) are a gross example of European fetishization of non-Western cultures. In the eyes of the art world, the styles that European artists appropriated were "primitive" or "naïve," but when imitated by Western artists, it was fine art.

Gender inequality kept women from having a place in the art world for centuries. The women's liberation movement in the 1960s brought about more change and opportunities for (mostly white) female artists to flourish, but even today, art made by women on average sells for much less than art made by men. In her essay "Why Is Work by Female Artists Still Valued Less Than Work by Male Artists?" the sociologist Taylor Whitten Brown points out a disheartening statistic that illustrates the sexism of the art world: "Only two works by women have ever broken into the top 100 auction sales for paintings, despite women being the subject matter for approximately half of the top 25."

In every creative industry — from fashion to filmmaking, from country music to the culinary arts — BIPOC, LGBTQ+ people, and women are paid less, lack representation, and have fewer opportunities than their white cis male counterparts. In addition, folks who fall under more than one of these groups—for example, being both Black and female—are faced with even greater challenges. This is not due to a lack of technical skill or talent, although marginalized people do have less access to art education and materials; it is due to an institution and industry still imprisoned by a thought system of Learned Hierarchical Beliefs, which tells us that not everyone's self-expression is valuable. The result? Our world has been robbed of experiencing the full spectrum of creative diversity. We have all been conditioned to see art through an internalized hierarchical lens—believing that in order to be artists and creators, we have to prove we are good enough.

But good enough for who, exactly?

Getting reacquainted with my inner weirdo.

One morning in my early twenties, I woke up totally hungover, to my partner saying something so bizarre that I thought I must still be dreaming.

"Let's make music together."

"What?"

"Let's make an album. You will be the vocalist and I will produce it."

I thought surely my partner wasn't thinking straight. At the time, we'd been together for a little over a year, and he had introduced me to the art scene in Williamsburg, Brooklyn. I had just graduated from college for acting and the highlight of my career was a Nickelodeon audition where the producer asked me to reread the lines and said, "This time actually act like you care." I had nothing going on.

The previous night, a few of his musician friends had come over to our apartment to make music and freestyle over some beats he made. To ease my social anxiety, I had taken some pretty large swigs of the tequila bottle everyone was passing around as I watched them take turns freestyling in the makeshift closet/recording booth. As the night went on, I got drunker and drunker. Before I knew it, I was in the booth.

"Check, check." I cringed hearing my voice on a microphone. It sounded like a mix of my mom's voice and a Teletubby's. Then the beat came in. *What am I gonna say? WTF am I doing?*

I closed my eyes and just let go. The words that came out of my mouth didn't make much sense and barely rhymed. I started saying I was a little bunny rabbit running around Brooklyn, and talked about eating carrots and burning down buildings, causing all kinds of havoc, and made strange rhythmic gibberish sounds to the beat — it was like an unhinged nursery rhyme. I don't know what came over me; I must have just been channeling my imagination. And it was unapologetically weird. When the beat ended and I came back to reality, I felt like I was going to throw up from embarrassment — or the tequila. Thank God they had been kind enough to clap.

And there we were the following morning and my partner was handing me a cup of coffee with this big grin on his face, the same one he had when I came out of the recording booth.

"Why would you want to make an album with me? I can't make music!" I said with a nervous laugh.

"Yes, you can. You went off last night, everybody loved it. It was so weird and so free. Come on, it will be cool. I'll be the producer and make the beats. You can be the front person and do the vocals. I already know what you should call yourself."

He was totally serious. I hadn't let loose like that around him, or anyone really, since I was little. Could I really make music? He seemed to think so. Maybe my weirdness, the part of me I'd worked so hard to conceal for fear of looking uncool, was actually cool?

"What should I call myself?" I asked him.

"Bunny Rabbit."

Having no experience or expectation made it easy for me to write and perform as Bunny Rabbit. I wasn't caught up in trying to be good, because I knew I wasn't traditionally good. We made music videos from our bedroom, sewed our own costumes, created sets from found trash, and got props from the dollar store for photoshoots. Everything was DIY because we had no other choice. But it was exciting. I had spent my college years trying to be the right kind of actor; as Bunny Rabbit, I didn't have to conform to a preconceived notion of what an artist was. For the first time, I didn't have to fit in, and it gave me the freedom to take up space.

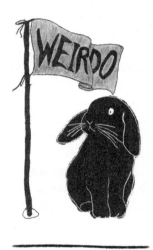

Your Creative Voice Matters

You are a channel for creative energy. It is the same creative energy that paints the flowers, grows the grass, and turns the acorn into an oak tree. You are part of nature, and when you choose to channel your creativity, it moves through you and comes out in forms shaped by your experience and perspective at that moment in time.

Everyone is an artist, but not everyone chooses to practice, because somewhere along the line, they started to believe it wasn't for them. But if everyone has a voice, a perspective, and an imagination, then being creative is a gift we can each express in our own unique way. That is why no two artists' work will be exactly the same. That is why the scribbly finger-painting you make in kindergarten is just as important as the painting you make in grad school. Both are a mirror to your Higher Self: revealing who you are beyond the limitations of what our world has dictated you are supposed to be. That is why art is so revolutionary and dangerous to an oppressive system. That is why a creative practice is so healing—because it is an affirmation that your perspective is meaningful, your voice matters, and that you are enough just for being you.

It's true that some people have a natural talent for certain artistic skills, but art is more than technical skill; it comes from somewhere deep within you. When other people's creativity inspires you, it touches on something that you also feel, even if you don't have a word for it—an experience you relate to, even if it didn't look the same. What you are drawn to is recognizing yourself in another person's creative voice. And in that way **art is an exchange of love**. The artist is saying, *I am you and you are me*. Let me show you another realm of experience of yourself and the world we live in. It saddens me to think about all the creative voices of previous generations that never had an opportunity to be heard, and all the creative voices of people today who have silenced that part of themselves out of fear of judgment or the belief that they aren't real artists.

LHBs Sabotage Self-Expression

Today, social media has revolutionized the ability we have to share our creativity and experience other creative voices. Still, many people struggle to accept that their creative expressions have value, and social media can exacerbate that insecurity by equating this value with likes. The key to a sustainable creative practice is recognizing that the number of people who connect to your art does not make it more or less valuable. If someone cannot recognize themselves in your work, they are simply in a different place in their journey and experience. That's all. Not liking a song or a movie or a painting simply means it's not for you. And that's why **you don't need an audience to receive the healing benefits of having a creative practice.** Similarly, having a large audience doesn't necessarily mean you are getting any healing benefit, especially if you are so focused on pleasing that audience that you lose touch with your Higher Self.

Artistic expression is the practice of accepting all the parts of yourself: joy, sorrow, confusion, ecstasy, anger...Art therapists understand that simply expressing your feelings through creative practice is healing because you are affirming those feelings as valid. Your Higher Self wants your art to show you that you are enough just how you are. When you use your art in service of your LHBs, however, you are putting a pressure on your creative expressions to make you whole; and just like any other relationship you put pressure on to complete you, your relationship to your creativity can become toxic.

I started seeking approval through my art.

"I can't believe you are calling yourself that."

My mom was standing in front of her kitchen counter, holding her coffee mug with two hands, as if keeping the cup level would also stabilize her emotions.

I was visiting my parents in Texas, fresh off a European tour for Bunny Rabbit. I had only spoken briefly to my parents about my new music career and thought they would be impressed by my international tour and the magazines I'd been featured in. I had just landed my first cover—which to me was a big deal—even if it was a magazine from the Netherlands and I had no idea what the article said because it was in Dutch. I couldn't wait for my mom to finally recognize that some people *actually liked* my quirky artistic nature. I imagined hearing

something along the lines of "I always knew you were special!" But the look on my mom's face sitting there in her kitchen
after I asked her what she thought of my music was reading as
totally pissed off.

"You can't believe I'm calling myself Bunny Rabbit? What is
wrong with that name? What are you talking about?" I asked.

"You know exactly what I'm talking about. I didn't raise you
that way," she said sharply.

My mom was looking at me with the same disapproving
glare she had given me in the car all those years ago — like she
was trying to figure out how she ended up with such a strange
daughter. A long silence filled the room.

Then it hit me. When my sisters and I were young, my mom
made up a word for our most private anatomical parts. It's what
a lot of parents do, probably to swaddle their children in a pro-
tective layer of innocence as if the words *vagina* and *penis* are
inherently dirty. *Bunny* was the word my mom used for vagina.
And now my mom thought that was exactly why I had chosen it
for a stage name. *Oh. My. God.*

I sat there dumbfounded. Could it be that on some unconscious level, calling myself a bunny rabbit in that freestyle had
been a nod to my sexuality, an artistically inspired Freudian
slip? Did she think I was intentionally desecrating a word that
symbolized a time when I was just her little girl, when I looked to
her for guidance and listened attentively when she explained
to me that only girls have bunnies? I had turned something
sacred into something strange and embarrassing. I thought,
*I guess Bunny is actually an appropriate name for me then,
because I am strange and embarrassing.*

That trip to Texas, along with the pressure I felt to keep making Bunny Rabbit successful, began to make me feel like what
I was making wasn't good enough. I thought if we were more
mainstream and landed a huge record deal, my parents and
everyone who ever doubted me would come around to being
proud of me instead. But **wanting more recognition meant**

focusing on what I didn't have. I started obsessing over how many online hits we got a day, what people said about me, and how I looked. I compared myself to other artists. When it came time to make new songs, I struggled with writing because channeling my imagination no longer seemed viable. It wasn't enough because *I* still wasn't enough. I was stuck in my LHBs, unable to see my own value as an artist without accumulating approval. On top of that, my partner's and my relationship had become extremely toxic. Before the second album was finished, we split up — and that was the end of Bunny Rabbit.

It would take years for me to understand that making art in order to fulfill a desire to be accepted *was* me losing my true artistic voice — the voice of my Higher Self. When you are trapped in your LHBs, you are stuck in the perspective of *lack*, because in order to feel successful you have to continually be more successful compared to other artists and creators. Your art practice is no longer about authentically expressing yourself — it becomes about "winning," and you forget why you loved making art in the first place. Learned Hierarchical Beliefs turn your creative passion into a weapon of self-loathing.

It's the nature of our careers and passions to have moments of growth and moments of difficulty. It's understandable to feel discouraged when things don't go the way you want. In order to sustain a healthy and joyful relationship with your creativity, you need to be clear on why you are doing it. Are you doing it to fulfill an unconscious sense of lack (LHB motivated), or are you doing it because you honor your self-expression and want to see where it takes you (Higher Self motivated)? One will lead you to sporadic, temporary bouts of happiness dependent on the approval of others, and the other will keep you grounded in the truth of your inherent worth and freedom to continue to create from your authenticity.

Creative Expression in Service to Love

When you are channeling your creativity, you are actively loving yourself, making you a more loving person to everyone you meet. When you know that the purpose behind your work is much more than wanting to be better than other people, or having more than other people, you will be able to receive the love your art is trying to give you. Creating art from the lens of your Higher Self is being in service to love.

Your creative expression is a blessing. It's an opportunity to explore your imagination, to share your deepest feelings, and to bring more beauty into your life. There is no right or wrong way to do it. But your Higher Self can empower you on your journey. Below are guidelines, journal prompts, and affirmations to help.

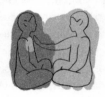

Harness the Power of Your Higher Self in Your Creative Practice

1. **Remember that your authentic self is your greatest creative asset.** People are inspired by authenticity because it makes them feel it is okay to be themselves. It's the most empowering place to be, both for the creator and for the witness. That doesn't mean you never make something that is similar to other people's work, because in many ways we are similar. It means that you will never run out of ideas, because you are

the main source of your inspiration, and there will never be a time in your life when you have nothing to say.

2. **Let go of the beliefs you have to be making money off your art to be an artist.** No matter what job is paying your bills, you are an artist. Your job, whether it's waiting tables, working at a bank, or selling your work in a gallery, is helping to keep your creative practice sustainable: It's paying for your studio, watercolors, acting classes, iPhone. Letting your job define who you are as an artist is putting your creative journey in the hands of an economic system based on Learned Hierarchical Beliefs. A system that doesn't reflect your value. When you use your creativity in service of your Higher Self, you help to dismantle that system and rebuild a world where all artists will have the means to create as much as they want, and where art is accessible to everyone. Do not let a capitalist system determine the value of your self-expression. It's invaluable.

3. **Stop judging the things you create so you can keep creating.** Being in a creative rut is an indication you are putting too much pressure on yourself to create something "good." When you create, you are channeling creative energy in the present moment, and if that present moment happens to produce something you think is shit, let it be shit. Who are you to say what the evolution of your creative journey should look like? That's like expecting every day of your life to be sunshine and rainbows. We all know that some of our worst days on this Earth have been our most transformative. It's the same for your art.

4. **Recognize the difference between jealousy and inspiration.** Jealousy is a product of a hierarchical thought system, believing that some people are better than others. Inspiration is receiving the gifts that another creator is offering you. Inspiration comes from *in-spirit* or in the consciousness of your Higher Self. Before you go to your friend's music show, or gallery opening, or log on to social media—pay attention to

what your motivation is. Is it to compare yourself to other artists, or is it to tap into the love that that artist is so courageously offering?

5. **Support and encourage other people's work.** Dismantling your Learned Hierarchical Beliefs about your art and creative practice means seeing other people's work from that lens as well. When you recognize the courage, beauty, and value in your peers' creations, it helps you to see that in your work, too. You are more powerful than you realize, and every time you give someone words of love and encouragement, you affirm their self-worth.

6. **If you don't like what someone makes, that doesn't mean there is anything wrong with it. It just means it's not for you.** I can think of a few music genres that never get played in my Spotify account. But there's no need to shout that from the rooftops. What a boring world it would be if we all liked the same things.

7. **You don't have to share your creativity with others (but if you want to, you should).** No matter who you are or what you make, not everyone is going to like it. When you share your work looking for validation, no amount is going to be enough. When you share it for the purpose of connecting to people on a deeper level, through your authentic voice, you are doing it for love. So before you make any decision to share, ask yourself *why*. Making art is an intimate experience with your Higher Self, and you don't have to share that with others in order for it to be valid.

LHBs About Creativity and Art vs. Your Higher Self

LHB: I shouldn't share my authentic creative self because I don't want to be judged.

Higher Self: Not sharing your authenticity means you are the one judging yourself.

LHB: I'm not an artist; I'm not getting paid for it.

Higher Self: Don't let a capitalist system determine the value of your self-expression. It's invaluable.

LHB: If my art was good then everyone would like it.

Higher Self: There is no such thing as good or bad art. There is only what you relate to and are inspired by. If someone doesn't like your art, it isn't for them.

Journal Prompts

1. My earliest memory of being creative/artistic is...

2. My fears about creativity are...

3. Beliefs about myself that contribute to those fears are...

4. Flip the script: What would your Higher Self say in response to those fears?

5. Some changes I could make in my behavior and/or routine to empower my creative practice are...

6. Some ways I could show more support to my fellow artists are...

7. Some ways I could reach out for more support from other artists are...

_____

8. My art is important because...

_____

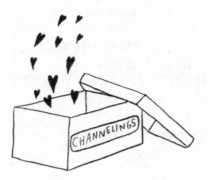

Exercise to Tap into Divine Creative Energy

1. Select your desired creative practice like writing, drawing, crafts, whatever you want. If you are singing or playing an instrument, prepare to record yourself on recording equipment or the voice memo app on your phone. If you are dancing, prepare to record a video of your dancing on your phone.

2. Dedicate a special place to store your art: For physical art like writing, drawing, and so on, get a folder or box you can store it in; if you are making a recording, making digital art, or writing on your computer, create a new folder on your computer. Label the storage "CHANNELINGS."

3. Dedicate one hour of uninterrupted time to "channel creative energy" by doing your practice without stopping and without caring what the outcome is or what it looks like or sounds like. In other words, do not try to make it "good." Let it pour

out of you no matter how it comes out. It can sound or look like total gibberish. The point is to keep going until the hour is done.

4. Take your writing, drawing, or recording and title it with to-day's date and put it away in your CHANNELINGS folder/box. Do *not* linger. Do not critique. Do not watch the recording or analyze the art. Put it away.

5. Do this as many days as you can for a full month. I'd recommend at least four days a week, if possible.

6. At the end of the month, you can watch/read/listen to your channelings. Notice what you find surprising or interesting about what you made. Notice what changes about your work the more uninhibited you feel. Do not share it with anyone. These channelings are for your eyes only. They are offerings to Divine Creative Energy. They are sacred.

7. Use them as inspiration moving forward. And if you ever feel stuck again, it's time for another channeling.

Chapter 3

Work and Productivity

> **Me:** *I've been dealing with so many feelings lately that I haven't been productive.*
>
> **Higher Self:** *What could be more productive than tending to your emotional well-being?*

We Were Taught Productivity Equals Self-Worth

The first time an adult asked me what I wanted to be when I grew up, I had no idea what they meant. *I have a choice in what I'm going to be? I thought I was going to be me.* Then I realized what they were asking was what I wanted to *do for work* when I grew up.

From the time we are very little, we get the message that what we choose to do for work is an essential, if not *the* most essential, part of who we are. We learn that it is important to have some idea of what we want to do before we leave high school—before our brains are fully developed. And we were encouraged to think this way by well-intentioned people who believed that in order to be respected, valued, and worthy, you must be productive. Your job is intrinsic to your identity, and the more productive you are, the more valuable you are to society and the more self-actualized you will be. And if you are not productive or willing to work hard enough, then you are labeled as lazy. Lazy people are a burden to society and morally flawed.

In his book *Laziness Does Not Exist,* Dr. Devon Price argues that the term "lazy" is a gross misrepresentation of the true barriers to the motivation and inspiration that allow people to have a healthy relationship to productivity. The myth of laziness, which he dubs the Laziness Lie, largely stemmed from productivity-obsessed forms of Christianity, and was used as justification for slavery and indentured servitude: If more work could improve a person's moral standing, it was believed, then forcing labor upon people was morally sound, even God's work. Likewise, the refusal to work was further proof of a person's inferiority.

The Learned Hierarchical Belief that *your productivity equals your worth* has caused generations of ableism and ageism bias—labeling people with disabilities or elderly people as a burden because they may not be able to contribute to the gross domestic product. Unemployed people are seen as second-class citizens. Poor people have no one else to blame but themselves.

Productivity LHBs are a founding principle of the American Dream—the idea that as long as you are productive, you are worthy of abundance and prosperity. If you don't work hard, then you have only yourself to blame for your financial hardships. By this logic, everyone working hard around the globe should be living comfortable and financially secure lives. But we all know that is very far from the truth.

Hard work was my family's love language.

I come from a lineage of extremely hardworking, productive people. My sisters and I heard stories growing up about my grandparents joining the influx of Mexican and Tejano migrant farm workers who traveled north every year to pick vegetables. We'd hear about how they raised their nine kids in a one-bedroom house, with my abuelito working two full-time jobs and my abuelita cooking dinner after long hours working at the meatpacking factory.

When I was a kid my abuelita was an intimidating person who wore her many years of hard work in a facial expression that read as *Make sure to stay out of the way.* She wasn't like the grandmas I'd see on TV spending quality time with their grandkids sharing Werther's Originals. The fruits of her labor, specifically the pork chops con chile and menudo she'd cook the entire extended family every Sunday, were her form of affection.

My dad had his own pull-yourself-up-by-your-bootstraps story. His high school counselor said he'd never make it in college because he was poor and Mexican, but he worked hard enough to prove the counselor wrong, eventually earning his master's degree even though there were days in college he didn't know where his next meal would come from.

And so it was with this expectation of an ingrained work ethic that at a young age my sisters and I helped our parents in the family business—an event production company that catered to the Mexican American community in Dallas, where we grew up. Our job was selling tacos and nachos during the Tejano music concerts and lowrider car shows they put on. During the summer we'd work all weekend outdoors, often in temperatures of 100 degrees or more. I remember coming home after an event weekend and collapsing on my bed, totally exhausted. We didn't just hear stories of hard work growing up; we learned through firsthand experience.

Despite the family business having years of success, around the time I was in middle school, it took a turn for the worse. I couldn't square how hard my parents were working with how much we were struggling to pay the bills. But what was worse than struggling with finances was seeing my parents so stressed out. It seemed like every time the business was failing, they thought *they* were failing. Often when I'd hear them arguing through the wall between their room and the one I shared with my two sisters, I'd fantasize about running in there screaming, "I don't care about money, I just want you to be happy!" And then they would have a huge epiphany, and smile and hug me and say something like, "You know, you are right, sweetheart." I think I saw something like that on an episode of *Full House*.

Eventually the family business came to an end, but not without its scars from the turmoil and stress of years of hard work and sacrifice. My dad told us if you work hard, then you can accomplish all of your dreams. And I'm so grateful that I had a parental figure that encouraged me even though I came to realize it's not that simple.

I don't love my parents because they worked hard; I love them for who they are. What I wanted more than anything else growing up was quality time with them, just being together. In his book, *The Myth of Normal: Trauma, Illness and Healing in a Toxic Culture*, the renowned physician and trauma expert Gabor Maté speaks extensively on the harmful effects that stress — including economic stress — in the home can have on child development, both emotionally and physiologically. But he is quick to point out that although it is commonplace to put all responsibility on the caregivers, what is missing is the acknowledgment of how difficult it is to raise children while living in a society with so much economic inequality and deprivation. "Yes, parents are responsible for their children; no, they did not create the world in which they must parent them."

As much as the story of my family's work ethic is a story of pride and resilience, it's also a story of loss. Loss of time spent together, loss of rest, loss of freedom. It's also a story of inequality, of sacrifice and pain. I don't want to romanticize their struggle. I want to honor it by acknowledging that it shouldn't have been that hard. I hope with all my heart during those difficult times they could hear their Higher Self reminding them how amazing, beautiful, and deserving they were and have always been, no matter the obstacles they faced.

The Illusion of "Self-Made"

Equating worth with productivity misleads people to think that a person's economic success is entirely reflective of their character. In this paradigm, if you don't make a lot of money, it's not due to the inequities of society, the circumstances of your environment, or your physical limitations — it's because you are lazy or not intelligent enough, or you didn't try hard enough. If you do have a lot of money, it has nothing to do with your privilege or luck; it's because you work harder or are smarter than other people.

When *Forbes* magazine put Kylie Jenner on their cover with the words "self-made billionaire" in 2019, people were rightly outraged by the oversimplification. How is she self-made when she comes from generational wealth? Popular culture's use of rags-to-riches stories has perpetuated the myth that a person's economic prosperity is entirely up to them. Two years later *Forbes* published a follow-up piece, claiming that the Jenner camp had likely falsified tax documents to make it look like Kylie had reached billionaire status in order to land their cover, when in reality she hadn't. While Jenner's representatives denied doing any such thing, it's easy to understand what would motivate people who were already rich and successful to feel they need to exaggerate their wealth even further in a culture where no amount of wealth is enough.

The truth is that no one is "self-made," because the success of any business is not solely determined by an owner's hard work. That myth disregards the labor of employees, the support of mentors, the financial benefits of investors, generational wealth, and the innovation of their creative influences. Not to mention, it discounts the barriers of race, class, sex/gender, and ableist discrimination that so many people face. According to a 2021 study, 46 percent of LGBTQ workers have experienced work discrimination, while four in five transgendered adults report that discrimination affects their ability to find work. Black and Latinx millennials earn fifty-four cents and sixty-four cents to every dollar of their white peers. When someone is seen as less valuable because of how they identify or their ancestral and/or economic background, they are seen as less deserving of livable wages and treated as if they have nothing of value to offer. LHBs create categories of superiority and inferiority, leading to dehumanization and suffering. Changing this system begins with acknowledging that everyone (including you) deserves to live in a society that supports their well-being because everyone has value.

It's Not the Avocado Toast

It's easy to be hard on ourselves when we are struggling with job security, starting our own business, or building a career. We had an image of what our lives would look like by the time we reached a certain age. We were told by older generations that our success was entirely up to us. Yet it's important to acknowledge the very real and unique challenges our generation faces—not so we throw in the towel and give up on our goals, but to be compassionate with ourselves and educated about the systems we are navigating. The fact is, things are not the same as they were for previous generations. College tuition has more than doubled since the 1980s, and healthcare costs are nine times higher than they were in the 1960s, even after being adjusted for inflation, yet wages and salaries have not kept up with these increased expenses. Millennials and Gen Z work longer hours than their parents despite making 20 percent less a year when factoring in inflation. Smartphones and email have made it harder to clock out.

Hustle culture, a contemporary take on the American Dream, is the idea that if you are really dedicated to something, you will work relentlessly at it, often sacrificing personal relationships and self-care. Overwork is glamorized all over the internet, from the YouTube influencer Gary Vaynerchuk saying that if you are excited about the end of a work week "you need to rethink your life," to Elon Musk tweeting that "nobody ever changed the world on 40 hours a week." But as David Heinemeier Hansson, the author of *It Doesn't Have to Be Crazy at Work,* points out, "The vast majority of people beating the drums of hustle-mania are not the people doing the actual work. They're the managers, financiers, and owners." And even though research suggests that longer hours do not increase a company's productivity, we continue to feel obligated to work longer for less pay and benefits.

Rather than putting energy into having compassion for ourselves and acknowledging the need for change in economic policies, we often blame ourselves and internalize any lack of success as an indicator that we are lacking. **The point isn't that determination and hard work are futile, it's that everyone needs help, support, encouragement, and opportunity.** And your Higher Self knows that is exactly what you and everyone else are warranted.

Punishing Ourselves with Productivity

When I was growing up, I was punished for not getting my chores done. Punishment was a strategy my parents used to teach me to do "better." They learned it from their parents. And their parents learned it from *their* parents. Many of us grew up that way. And now we use self-punishment as a misguided form of self-improvement. Of course, most of us don't spank ourselves or ground ourselves or force ourselves into time-out—no, our way of self-punishment comes in packages like mentally putting ourselves down, telling ourselves we are failures, refusing to acknowledge our accomplishments and self-worth, denying ourselves rest, and feeling like we don't deserve joy and pleasure unless we are sufficiently productive.

A lot of us were raised in homes where we were made to feel that no matter what we did, it was never enough to be loved. Maybe you were neglected as a child, abused, or mistreated. If this is the case, productivity and accomplishment can feel like the answer to finally becoming lovable, respected, admired, and accepted. Work becomes an avenue not only for earning money but for earning self-worth.

If you believe your worth is equal to your productivity, shame and guilt will be your primary sources of motivation. This is because on a fundamental level you feel you are lacking, and that being as productive as possible will take away that feeling of lack. Everything you cross off your to-do list becomes a small step toward being okay with yourself. But the to-do list is never completed. It's like you are always swimming in a current, struggling to keep your head above water, and each accomplishment grants you just a couple of breaths.

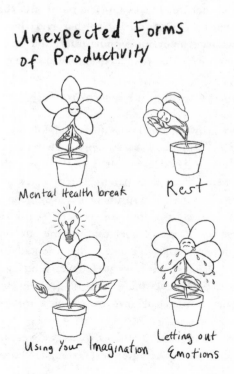

Unexpected Forms of Productivity

Mental Health break

Rest

Using Your Imagination

Letting out Emotions

Our lack of compassion when it comes to our own productivity and our culture's overzealous individualism prevents us from helping others or asking for help when we need it. The only way for us to change our culture's understanding of work and productivity is to understand what we deserve as human beings and to demand better for ourselves and for each other.

You Are So Much More Than Your Output

From the Higher Self perspective, you were born worthy, you were born whole, and you do not need to prove that to yourself or to others. You deserve to have a life that is reflective of your inherent value. Every one of us is a gift to this world. And when we remove the lens of our LHBs and see that our productivity does not equal our value, we can start making choices motivated by our Higher Selves, not our fear of lack. Rest, recuperation, self-care, processing emotions, and even doing nothing are just as valuable as answering emails. In order to live a life reflective of how worthy you already are, you need to take care of yourself. When you work from love, from the perspective of your Higher Self, you are more in touch with your passions, with what inspires you, and with your creativity, because you are tapped into the value of your own perspective and experience. You advocate for compassionate work environments for yourself and others. You understand that you are part of a whole. Bringing to light the cultural and personal narratives that contribute to your fears of unworthiness will empower you in your relationship with work and productivity and will also help you have compassion for the people around you who are also struggling with similar fears.

Let's say, for example, that there has been a managerial change at work, and your new boss has been treating you unkindly. Their attitude has also created a hostile and toxic work environment, and you internalize their treatment as stemming from failure on your part. Because you are not conscious of your Higher Self, you are used to equating your value with how well you are doing at your job. In this case, not only is having a work "superior" put you down very hard on you, but you are at a loss as to what to do about it. You feel discouraged and unhappy. You fear further criticism and are anxious and on edge. So you keep your head down to avoid your boss's wrath. Then when you come home from work, you are upset, angry, and exhausted. The more time you spend at that job, the more it wears you down.

When you are in the consciousness of your Higher Self, however, you realize that your boss is just another person who is also on the journey of realizing their own self-worth. Someone who has most likely been treated unfairly by a work superior themselves, because toxic work environments are a product of a hierarchical culture that equates human value with productivity. You realize that your boss's inability to be kind has nothing to do with how worthy you are of that kindness. And the first thing that has to change is the belief that somehow your boss's behavior is your fault. After that, you can decide if looking for another job with a healthier work environment or advocating for better treatment at your current job will be the best way to move forward.

When you acknowledge how worthy you are of compassion, care, and abundance, you can be clear about what choices and what environments will sustain your journey to self-love. When you put pressure on your work to define your value, even if you are doing what you love, you will find it very difficult to create boundaries that support your well-being.

Work and productivity are a part of your experience on this planet, but they do not define who you are. When you are able to separate your identity from your job, you can have a much clearer perspective on that job. Am I being treated fairly? What is my state of consciousness at work? What am I really passionate about? Am I getting enough rest? Do I need to ask for help? When you equate work with your worth, you lose perspective. Career paths are up and down. Other people's choices are out of your control. What *is* in your control is knowing your inherent value, advocating for yourself, and making choices about your work and productivity that reflect your value.

I had to learn how to rest.

"You know, Bunny, you don't have to feel bad to take a break."

My spouse interrupted the episode of *Dateline* I was watching while snuggled under a blanket on our couch with my cat, Pepper, purring heavily next to me. The past few days, I had been working frantically to finish a deadline, but an hour ago my body started aching; when I came downstairs to complain to Khara, they suggested I take the rest of the day off. So I turned on the TV and got under a blanket.

And then right before the moment Keith Morrison was about to reveal the verdict of a suburban housewife accused of poisoning her husband with antifreeze for insurance money, Khara began insinuating that I was not actually feeling unwell.

"What do you mean, you don't think I feel bad?" I shot back.

"No, I'm just saying that you never let yourself rest simply because you need rest. But you should. Everyone needs rest," they responded with a warm smile.

My spouse does this thing that really annoys me. They tell me things that I spend most of my time telling other people to do. Like to be nice to myself, or that I need self-care, or to stop calling myself stupid. And it annoys me because I know they are right. My LHBs about productivity are some of my most difficult ones to unlearn. No matter how much I work, it's a challenge for me to feel like I am doing enough. And I know a lot of that comes from my grandparents and my parents, who were forced into circumstances that required them to go nonstop. I didn't grow up with an example of self-care. I thought I wasn't allowed to take a break if there were still things that needed to be done. And I never wanted to disappoint my dad, who told me that all I have to do is believe in myself.

But in my heart, I know that believing in myself isn't working harder than anyone else; it's knowing that despite the ups and downs of career success, I am valuable and worthy of abundance. And that I deserve to live in a world where everyone is treated that way.

I flashed my spouse a knowing smile and realized that my body aches weren't as strong as before. For a moment I thought, *I should get back up and work again*. But instead I asked Khara if they would go to the kitchen and make me a cup of hot cocoa with extra marshmallows.

Work as a Path to Healing

We live in a world that is heavily influenced by LHBs about productivity. But change comes from the inside and reverberates outward. When you become more aware of your LHBs about productivity, your work becomes an avenue to awaken and heal. It doesn't matter if you are a therapist or a barista or a stay-at-home mom with four kids — bringing your Higher Self to the work you do infuses that work with the consciousness of love. Everyone you touch, work with, come in contact with, feels that on some level. And the result is a completely different energy and often inspires healing in the people around you as well. We are part of a collective awakening to our Higher Selves, and you shifting your beliefs is a seed to our shared blossoming. Work does not give you meaning; you give meaning to your work by letting it teach you how to more fully love and care for yourself.

Bringing your Higher Self to your work and productivity is a practice. Do not judge yourself if it feels really difficult right now — everything is difficult when you are not used to it! Here are some guidelines, affirmations, and journal prompts to help get you started.

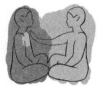

Bring Your Higher Self to Your Work

1. **Remember you are not your work, even if you love your work.** From an early age, you were conditioned to believe that *what you do* is *who you are*. This is so far from the truth! You are a divine, creative, compassionate, inspired, empathetic, curious, open-hearted, beautiful being. Who thinks, feels, imagines, fantasizes, loves, cares, cries, yells, sings, dreams, kisses, hugs, teaches, learns, grows, and is on a journey of awakening. There is so much more to you than what you do to pay your bills.

2. **Define what productivity means to you.** Is rest productive? Is going to therapy productive? Is taking a day off productive? It's all about how you look at it. You know that when you are well rested and taking care of yourself, you are more focused and present in all aspects of your life, including your work. Some of my strongest creative ideas have come to me when I'm taking a break from working on my art.

3. **Ask for help.** Being raised in a productivity-obsessed culture makes you feel like you should be able to do everything on your own. The myth of the self-made hero makes it seem like all you need to meet your goals is determination. But the

truth is, everyone needs help. Everyone needs inspiration. Everyone needs support. Everyone needs opportunity. And everyone deserves it. If you are used to doing things all on your own, asking for help can seem scary. It can even seem like you are admitting failure. But it actually means you care enough about yourself to know that you don't have to do it all alone.

4. **Expecting yourself to always feel motivated to be productive is unrealistic.** Hey, guess what? You're not supposed to always feel motivated to work and be productive, because you are not meant to always be working or being productive! You are not a machine!

5. **Laziness is a myth.** The next time you feel lazy, remember that laziness is a Puritanical myth based on the sin of idleness used to oppress people into forced labor. You either need more rest or more inspiration, or are denying yourself what you want because a part of you feels like you don't deserve it.

6. **Shame and guilt are not sustainable motivators for self-improvement.** If you're reading this book, you are probably interested in holding yourself accountable, but accountability is not the same as shame and guilt. Shame and guilt perpetuate low self-worth, leading to beliefs that you don't deserve to be happy, healthy, and fulfilled. If you have a goal you want to reach or something you want to get done, encouragement, compassion, kindness, and love are your superpowers. Imagine talking to a child and trying to get them to do something. You could shame or scare them into it, or motivate them by telling them how amazing they are. Shame might work once or twice, but eventually it will lead to resentment, anger, and sadness. Love from your Higher Self is the best form of motivation.

7. **Keep in mind that the people you work with have LHBs, wounds, and insecurities just like you.** Work relationships — whether it's with your boss, employees, or coworkers — aren't always easy to navigate. When you stay mindful that everyone

is in a different stage of awakening to their self-worth, it's easier to not take things personally when someone does something you feel is disrespectful or unprofessional. That doesn't mean you don't take action or advocate for yourself; it means you know that their behavior is not an indication that you are not worthy of healthy work environments. Additionally, connecting to your Higher Self also helps you have more patience, kindness, and respect for your coworkers, because you see the humanity in them and know that is what they deserve.

Work and Productivity Affirmations

- Whatever I am doing right now would be a lot easier if I was being nice to myself.
- Life is hard enough. I don't need to be hard on myself.
- I will stop judging myself for not being at a place in my life I thought I would be by this age. I am enough right now.
- I can ask for help because my Higher Self knows I deserve it.
- I don't have to earn rest.
- I trust my path and the future is bright.

Journal Prompts

1. The beliefs I learned growing up about work and productivity are...

   _____

2. In what ways have those beliefs been helpful? In what ways were they harmful?

   _____

3. The thoughts I'd like to shift about my relationship to productivity are...

    _____

4. Flip the script: The ways my Higher Self would respond to the above thoughts are...

    _____

5. Changes (if any) in my behavior and/or environment that will help me connect to my Higher Self more often when I am working are...

    _____

Chapter 4

Money and Abundance

Me: *The more I have, the more I am.*
Higher Self: *You have always been all you need to be.*

Growing up, I always wanted what my friends had.

Lindsay's mom's hands were thin, delicate, and the color of a peach Crayola. From the back seat of her Lexus, I could see her diamond ring twinkle as she turned the wheel, driving me home. It was my first time playing at Lindsay's house after school, and I couldn't wait to tell my sisters that she had two living rooms (one with white carpet we weren't allowed to walk on), a piano, a pool, and a trampoline. But I was most in awe of her giant pantry with boxes of every snack you could want: Dunkaroos, Zebra Cakes, Gushers…you name it. When

Lindsay told me to pick something, I went for the box of Fruit by the Foot.

"You can't have those, they are for my brother." She pointed to his name written on the box. I noticed every box was labeled with "Lindsay" or "Blake."

"You don't share?" I asked.

"No," said Lindsay with a proud smirk.

"Oh." I couldn't imagine having a box of snacks in the pantry that I didn't have to share with my sisters.

"Here, have a Nutter Butter, that's what I am having."

I didn't have the guts to tell Lindsay that I didn't like Nutter Butters. I didn't want to seem ungrateful.

The car ride home felt so smooth, like the tires were made of marshmallow fluff. The leather seats were almost the same peach Crayola color as Lindsay and her mom. They reminded me of the chameleon lizards we had just learned about in science class that blend in to their environment.

"So, how was your summer? Did your family go on any vacations?"

Vacation? My summer consisted of staying home with my sisters, watching *The Price Is Right, Family Feud,* and *Oprah,* drinking Kool-Aid, and making sure our chores were done before our parents got home from work. Lindsay, like most of the other kids in my fifth grade class, went to summer camp and vacation. I could feel my throat getting tight, trying to think of what to say.

"Yes, we went on vacation," I lied. "We went to Hawaii."

"Oh wow, that's great. We went to Hawaii a couple of years ago, didn't we, Lindsay? What island did you go to?"

Uh-oh.

"What...island? Um, we went to...all of them."

"Oh, wow, how lovely!"

"You can turn right here," I said when we approached the sign for Preston Bend Apartments. Lindsay's mom slowed down but stopped short of turning in.

"You live in *these* apartments?" she asked.

"Yes."

Lindsay and her mom gawked at the bluish-gray building as the Lexus inched through the parking lot like we were on some not-fun version of *It's a Small World* at Disneyland.

There's this weird thing that happens when adults feel sorry for you. Their tone changes. Their smile gets bigger. And they say things they don't mean.

"Oh, I pass by these apartments all the time, but I haven't seen them up close. They are just lovely."

Finally, when we reached my apartment, I thanked them and raced inside so they would stop looking at me. I flopped on the living room couch and thought about what Lindsay would think if she came over. Would she still believe I went to Hawaii? Would she still want to be my friend? *Maybe it's better if I don't invite her over,* I decided. *I don't think she will want to blend in here.*

The Haves and the Have-Nots

Growing up, it didn't take long before we got the message that the more you have, the better you are. Pop culture fed us images of happy sitcom families living in nice houses, and glorified the lives of the rich and famous. Commercials were constantly selling us on the newest toy, with the happiest-looking kids playing with them. Soon we began noticing how our families measured up financially compared to our peers at school—how big was our house compared to theirs? How many presents did you get over the holidays? Brands of clothes and shoes became markers of status.

If you grew up in a home where you couldn't afford what your peers had, it was easy to internalize that as an inadequacy. *Why doesn't my family have what they have? What's wrong with us?* If you grew up in a home where you didn't know where your next meal was coming from, money represented instability and anxiety.

Some of you grew up in homes where money wasn't a source of economic insecurity but was used in place of intimacy and quality time, with caregivers supplementing their reduced presence with material gifts. Some of you grew up with expectations that when you reached adulthood you must achieve monetary success in order to receive approval.

Even if your caregivers taught you compassion, gratitude, and generosity, you still got the cultural message that the more you had the more you are.

I'm not here to say that money has nothing to do with happiness. Without financial security, people struggle to survive. Everyone needs and deserves to live economically safe lives. But there is a difference between needing money and the belief that people that have more are better than you.

This Learned Hierarchical Belief that the more you have, the more you are, makes us feel like failures when we struggle financially. Likewise, it promises that making more money will boost your self-worth. But your Higher Self knows that the number in your bank account does not define you. And when you attach your self-worth to that number, no amount will be enough, because according to your LHBs, you need to be in constant pursuit of more because you are fundamentally lacking.

Inner Abundance

You are inherently abundant. You are full of love. You were created whole.

Your Higher Self knows that what you bring to the table — your talents, your perspective, your creativity, your dedication, your commitment, your integrity, and your time — is valuable. You deserve to be compensated fairly and so does everyone else. Aligning with your Higher Self helps you avoid making financial decisions based on the desire to be validated through material wealth.

And it helps you to stop making assumptions that you are incapable of making more money or that you're undeserving of money, resources, and care when you are unable to work. You acknowledge that yes, this world isn't set up with equal opportunity, but that doesn't make you less equal—it inspires you to demand better for yourself and for humanity. It helps you see creative solutions and become part of communities that are supporting those in need. It motivates you to educate yourself about your rights, where your tax money is going, how the economy you live in actually works, and how to advocate for change.

Every human being deserves to live in an environment that reflects their wholeness. There are enough resources on this planet for every person to not have to struggle to meet their needs. But for generations upon generations we have not been taught our inherent self-worth—our inner abundance—and have been misguided into seeking that worth outside of ourselves. It doesn't have to be this way.

Going Deeper

So how do we change this? It's understandable to believe capitalism is to blame for how entrenched our hierarchical beliefs are when it comes to money and possessions. If we just got rid of an economic system where greedy CEOs and corporations with power-hungry politicians in their pockets get to trample on people with less power in the name of competition, then we wouldn't struggle with believing our self-worth is tied to the number in our bank accounts.

But that doesn't go deep enough. Greed stems from the vicious cycle of a system that tells people they are not good enough but they *could* be if they just possessed more—yet continuing to accrue possessions only leads to a deeper void, and the search continues. Individuals being conditioned by their LHBs try to fill the void of low self-worth with more money, more possessions, and when that isn't enough, they seek power and dominance over other people.

Greed attempts to satisfy the illusion that having more than other people makes you a more worthy human being.

Until we realize that no one is worthier than anyone else, there will always be some form of seeing other people through the lens of hierarchical beliefs and there will always be those who suffer because of it. It isn't just structural economic change that needs to happen but a change in the belief system that motivates that structure. Without our Higher Selves, we won't be able to create a world where everyone is valued. Until we awaken to our inherent worth and the worth of all human beings, all of us will make choices based on the illusion of lack. And we are all susceptible to causing harm because of it.

Greed is a consequence of believing the false promise that you are essentially lacking and will be complete only if you have more than other people. In reality, focusing on exterior factors with a comparison mindset will keep you trapped in feelings of inadequacy, not free you from them. You will never experience true abundance if you don't understand your true value. Not because you are better than other people, but because you realize the hierarchy of human worth is an illusion. An illusion that creates suffering.

I had to let go of shame.

For years I avoided thinking about money out of shame. Even after I took out a student loan for college, I avoided thinking about money. Sometimes I would avoid checking my account balance because logging in to the bank website gave me anxiety. I avoided budgeting because then I had to think about money even more. I didn't know how to begin saving. I worked my job, and I paid my rent. After college I deferred my student loans. I paid for food and clothes on credit cards with huge interest rates, which ended up in collections. The more debt I incurred, the more shame I felt, and the more shame I felt, the less I wanted to face my debt.

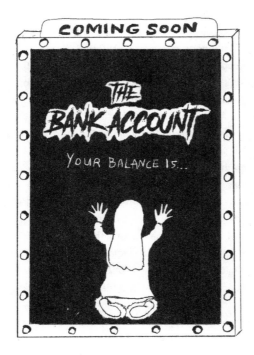

In my thirties, I turned to self-help and spiritual books that introduced concepts like manifesting financial abundance, or using the law of attraction (the idea that positive thinking would lead to positive things happening in your life) to have more money. I'd feel hopeful for a short time until it didn't seem to be working for me, which led me to believe that I wasn't strong or spiritual enough to make that happen, which led to more shame.

As I slowly became more connected to my Higher Self, doing the daily practice of writing my Higher Self memes, I started to shift my relationship to money by becoming more aware of the LHBs I was holding on to. I realized that a lot of my fear around money came from memories of being a young child and feeling out of control, unable to do anything to help my parents. Connecting to my Higher Self helped me realize that I am no longer that scared child, and that those experiences do not define me. Nor are they anything to be ashamed about. **Struggling financially is not an indication that you are failing—it's an indication that you need more support, inspiration, guidance, and opportunity.**

Acknowledging my LHBs helped me see my economic situation more clearly: Our financial system is based upon inequality, and it is set up to make certain demographics feel as though they don't deserve access to the education or guidance they need to make that system work for them—and I was holding on to shame for not having that knowledge. I wasn't inadequate because of my struggle; I was simply working with what I knew and the experience I had. I stopped blaming myself. I started acknowledging the challenges of making money while at the same time understanding that there are a lot of resources in the world and that I deserve access to them just as much as anyone else.

I started educating myself on the terms of my debts, my expenses, and my goals. I started keeping track of my spending, and brainstorming creative ways to monetize my art in addition to waiting tables, starting with crowdfunding from my community and supporters, applying for grants, and figuring out how to turn my art into merchandise I could sell. With every small step toward addressing my finances, I was silencing that voice in my head from childhood, the voice that said I would always be less-than. It was scary, anxiety-inducing, and triggering, but I kept reminding myself that my financial situation was not a test of my value, and slowly I stopped treating it like it had the power to make me or break my spirit.

Most important, connecting to my Higher Self helped me realize that healing my relationship to money was so much more than the ability to manifest it. It was about getting really clear as to what beliefs were motivating that desire—is it my LHBs, or is it that my Higher Self knows I am worthy of support, guidance, and living a life that is reflective of my inner abundance?

Expanding Gratitude

The concept of gratitude is used a lot in self-help and spiritual rhetoric. But often I feel we need to expand our approach to gratitude on not just what you have but who you are. Being grateful for who you are grounds you in your Higher Self. When you don't acknowledge your inner abundance, you start to see everything around you through that lens of lack. You can't "count your blessings" without acknowledging that you yourself are a blessing. Rather than approaching gratitude from what is outside of you, think about it as a shift in your consciousness to being aware of your wholeness within, then reflecting that abundance outward. When you give yourself love, you will see how full of love your life really is.

Get Out of Your Own Way

When you think about the economic disparities in the world, or your student loan debt, or whether or not you can afford to pay your phone bill, it can feel very overwhelming. It's easy to get discouraged. But too often we don't see how our LHBs keep us stuck in a cycle of cynicism and low self-worth, and capitalism profits when you feel lacking. A hierarchical system also depends on people feeling complacent to maintain the status quo. It needs you to feel disempowered and unmotivated, because that way you won't start to demand better for yourself. Accessing your Higher Self gives you courage to step out of your comfort zone and into the realization you can change your life. You are your Higher Self and you are more powerful and capable than your LHBs would have you think.

Being empowered by your Higher Self does not mean your LHBs are not going to come up. We live in a world that is organized around LHBs. So that is to be expected. Our childhood experiences with money are very impactful. So those narratives don't easily go away. The point isn't to totally get rid of those thoughts, but to begin questioning them. Who is speaking when I tell myself I'll never make enough money? Who put that thought in my head that says I'm not good enough unless I have a bigger house or more expensive clothes? What belief has led me to think that I don't deserve support when I need it? Over time those thoughts become less powerful. They don't influence all of your choices. They don't steal your joy. You are internally abundant. You are capable, wise, and compassionate. You can do this.

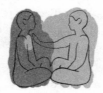

Bring Your Higher Self into Your Relationship with Money and Abundance

1. **Investigate the narratives you grew up with around money.** It's no secret that childhood experiences have a huge influence on our perspective. But often we don't apply that to our views around money. We tend to think our perspective is the correct one, even if it disempowers us. Sometimes even well-intentioned parental figures tell us things that aren't helpful, like "Money is the root of all evil" or "You need to buy a house by the time you are thirty." Think about your preconceived notions about money and ask yourself, *Is this helpful or harmful?*

2. **Empower yourself with financial literacy.** I don't know about you, but I was well into my adulthood before I understood what financial terms such as "interest rate," "Roth IRA," or "401k" meant. Our education system left us pretty unprepared to navigate a confusing economy. In my experience, most of the people raised with financial education come from families with generational wealth. But it's never too late to learn! There is so much information online, now including YouTube videos and online workshops. Don't be intimidated if you're new to all this—everyone starts somewhere.

3. **Do not put yourself down for your past choices.** Who hasn't looked back at their past financial decisions and felt the pain of regret (for example, taking out tens of thousands of dollars of student loan debt when you were just seventeen and really didn't understand how that debt would affect your future)? It's difficult to look back and think, *I wish I had known better.* You are not the sum of your past decisions. You were working with what was available to you in terms of education and self-awareness. This stuff isn't easy. Give yourself grace and take it one day at a time.

4. **Be generous when you can.** Our culture raised us to think that whatever you give, you lose. But from the Higher Self perspective, giving to others is also a gift to yourself, because it is an acknowledgment that what you give does not take away from your worth. If you are able to be generous with your finances, please do. Even the smallest extras can make someone feel really good. I remember when I waited tables, especially on busy days, when someone would add an extra few bucks on the tip, it would really brighten my day because I felt seen and appreciated. Also, there are many ways to be generous that aren't in the form of money. It can be giving your time, giving a compliment, giving a homemade gift, cooking someone a meal...the list goes on and on. Acts of generosity are expressions of love from your Higher Self.

5. **Acknowledge your blessings.** It almost feels cliché to suggest writing a list about what you are grateful for, but honestly, you should write a list of what you are grateful for. It's a life hack to seeing abundance instead of lack. Just because you feel grateful doesn't mean you can't want or desire other things. You can feel both!

Affirmations

- I embrace my inner abundance. I am worthy of bringing more abundance into my life.
- Whatever I am going through right now is a lesson in accepting myself. *All* of myself. Even the things I am working on changing. There is nothing wrong with me. There never was.
- I can change my relationship to money.
- I can ask for help and I can seek out guidance.
- It's never too late to learn about finances.
- I am a blessing to my own life.
- There is a lot of wealth and resources in this world and I deserve access to both as much as anyone else does.
- I can be generous because I have a lot of love to give.
- My Higher Self guides my financial decisions.
- I believe in my capacity to change my financial situation for the better. I am worth the effort.

Journal Prompts

1. My fears about money are...

_____

2. The experiences and/or cultural conditioning that have contributed to that fear are...

_____

3. Some of my negative perspectives around money and
    abundance are...

    _____

4. Flip the script: My Higher Self would respond to each of
    those negative thoughts with...

    _____

5. I am worthy of abundance because...

    _____

6. Changes in my behavior and/or steps I can take to empower
    my Higher Self around my finances are...

    _____

7. Ways that I can be more generous in my life are...

    _____

Chapter 5

Family and Childhood

"If you think you're so enlightened, go spend a weekend with your parents."

—Ram Dass

"Come on, we are almost there," said my sister Felili as we walked in the sweltering Texas heat. Felili was twelve years old, I was nine, and Maria, the youngest, was six. It was summer break and Felili was taking care of us while our parents were at work, like she did every summer. She was in charge of making sure we were fed and did our chores. She would come up with activities for us to do so we didn't just watch TV all day, like arts and crafts. She taught Maria how to read before kindergarten. When our parents had to work late, she made us dinner.

Felili had a hard time making friends because she had so many responsibilities at home and our mom was strict. When she got invited to the birthday party sleepover of a girl in her fifth-grade class, Mom wouldn't let her spend the night. Felili cried and begged, but of course Mom said no. Dad picked her up from the party while all the other girls got to stay. When she came home, I felt so sad for her, I gave her the rest of my strawberry Nerds.

On that particular summer day, Felili had the idea for the three of us to walk to the rec center by our school, like a mini field trip. It was about one mile from our apartment complex, but with the nearly 100-degree weather, it might as well have been on the other side of the earth. It felt like we were in the *Oregon Trail* computer game, where all the family members eventually die from heat stroke or dysentery before reaching California.

When we finally arrived at Campbell Green rec center and opened the front door, a wave of frigid AC collided with our overheated sweaty bodies, like when you put ice cubes in a warm glass of Kool-Aid and a little smoke floats out of the top. I could hear the screeching of sneakers from the boys playing basketball as we headed straight to the back and reached the apex of our journey—the vending machines.

Felili took some change from her pocket. We had just enough money for one Welch's grape soda and one bag of cherry sours. Then the three of us sat down on the cool gym floor and took turns having sips after dividing the candy into three equal portions.

"When we get home, we need to start our chores," Felili said, barely giving us a moment to relax. "Mel, it's your turn to clean the kitchen."

Meeting our parents' approval in terms of our responsibilities and behavior was a palpable pressure my sisters and I felt growing up. In my elementary school years my parents were often stressed out about work, so there was always a feeling we were walking on eggshells. Not meeting an expectation or "talking back" could be the catalyst for outbursts of anger and punishment from my mom. On top of that, we weren't allowed to do much outside the home. My mom's default answer for us going to a friend's house while they were at work was no. On the weekends when she was home, our days were filled with more responsibilities, like laundry and scrubbing the bathroom. Whether or not we were going to have a good day often hinged on my mother's mood. It felt extremely easy to disappoint her and to feel responsible for her unhappiness.

My dad's way of coping with stress and our mom's emotional shifts was to play it totally cool, with the outlook that everything was always "fine" and that there was nothing to worry about, no matter how bad things got. My dad's denial of anything being wrong at home, combined with my mother's emotional outbursts, made me feel like there was no safe place to talk about or process the instability I was feeling.

Although I have many happy memories from childhood and knew my parents loved me, the level of stress and uncertainty in our home for certain time periods was painful to experience. The more unhappy my parents were and the more anger and frustration my mom took out on us, the less deserving of love, kindness, and affection I often felt.

The first time I talked about my childhood with a therapist, I felt angry and confused. I would walk out of the therapist's office in Manhattan at the end of the session, head straight for a bar on Sixth Avenue, and down two shots of whiskey (this was before I learned healthier coping skills). Soon after I began working with my therapist, I started to connect how my childhood experiences had led to unhealthy patterns in my behavior and relationships as an adult. But even after those realizations, I felt something was missing. Just becoming more conscious of that stuff didn't make me feel any better. In fact, it made me more upset, because for years I had tucked all that stuff away so I wouldn't have to think about it. But as I began to confront it, it was all I could think about. Spending time with my family got harder, not easier. I was angry. I was hurt. I kept asking myself, "So now what do I do? How do I move past this?"

Uncovering Your Story

It's no big secret that the relationships you had with your family growing up have a huge effect on how you see yourself today. These relationships were your first examples of love, boundaries, communication, and nurturing—no matter how healthy or toxic they were. And uncovering how those dynamics have shaped your behavior and self-image is no easy process. It takes courage to go there.

When we begin seeing how our childhood experiences have influenced our adult behaviors and self-image, it can be overwhelming. We uncover resentment, insecurity, and anger. We observe the same toxic behaviors in our romantic relationships that our caregivers showed us. We realize we never learned to advocate for our boundaries when we have come from homes where our boundaries were constantly crossed. We became codependent or people pleasers when love was withheld from us as kids, or we felt we had to sacrifice our own needs to be lovable. We learned to dissociate from difficult emotions because that was our coping strategy for the trauma we experienced growing up. No matter who you are or where you came from, no one had a perfect childhood. No one had perfect parents. No one had every need perfectly met by their caregivers.

You Are So Much More than Your Story

No matter what stage you are in, when it comes to addressing your childhood wounds, the key to healing isn't just to uncover that stuff and connect the dots—it's to shift your identification from the story of your past to the story of your deeper truth—your Higher Self.

Often people ask me, "How do I let go of the past?"

The past was an experience. You don't have to let go of an experience. *You just have to let go of believing that that experience defines you.*

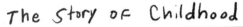

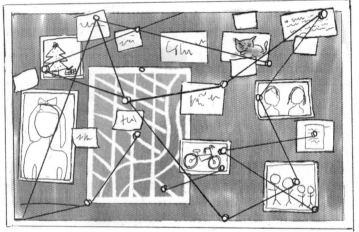

Your Higher Self is who you are *beyond* your conditioning, beyond what society defines you as. It's who you are beyond the predetermined expectations of your parental figures about how you were supposed to behave, what you should look like, what was worthy of punishment and what was worthy of reward, what part of you elicited love and attention and what elicited scorn and rejection. You were born into an environment of adults who already had their own LHBs about things like gender, body image, materialism, classism, homophobia, and white supremacy. They had already been living in a world that functions around Learned Hierarchical Beliefs. Not to mention they also had wounds and trauma of their own.

And then you arrived—pure, openhearted, unashamed, curious, without bias or hatred, never questioning that you deserved care. You were born fully embodied in your Higher Self—into an environment that to varying degrees slowly began to shut out that light.

It's not all your caregivers' responsibility. They were also born into an environment where their Higher Selves weren't necessarily supported or even seen. Even if they came from upbringings of compassionate acceptance and love, they were still part of a society that told them they needed to prove their worth.

When we think of family, we don't necessarily think about how LHBs have affected such intimate parts of our lives. How patriarchy, racism, social injustice, economic oppression, and other hierarchical structures might have played a role in our family's dysfunction. Rather, we internalize our difficult childhood experiences and our trauma as an inadequacy.

If I am really lovable, then I wouldn't have been treated that way. If I am worthy of acceptance, then I would have been accepted by my family. I will always be a wounded person because of my childhood wounds. I won't be able to have healthy relationships because I grew up around unhealthy ones. I cannot approve of myself because I never received approval from my parents. If I was normal, then I would have had a normal family. We believe the more things that were "wrong" about our childhood, the more possibility that something is wrong with us.

Letting go of those personal narratives takes seeing your situation through the lens of your Higher Self—LHBs are passed down generationally. If you were wounded by a family member or suffered a form of neglect or loveless behavior, it isn't because you are unlovable. It is because of their limitations in knowing how to love you, not your limitations in deserving that love.

My Higher Self connected the dots.

The more I connected to my Higher Self, the more I was able to see my family members through that lens, too. I was able to acknowledge that like me, they have wounds, trauma, and unconscious Learned Hierarchical Beliefs.

I began to see them beyond the role they played in my childhood, as individuals on their own journey. Which freed me to let go of the role I played with them.

My mom was born in American Samoa, an island with a culture that, since the arrival of missionaries in the 1830s, had become a mix of both dogmatic Christianity and indigenous Fa'a Samoa tradition — "a complex cultural code that guides and teaches individuals on how to lead their life," which has been part of Polynesian culture for three thousand years. Fa'a Samoa (which translates as "the Samoan way") puts a heavy emphasis on family obligation. Every member is expected to contribute to the success of the family.

When my mom was four years old, her parents moved the family to Hawaii for more opportunity and a better education. My mom and her twelve siblings were raised to be dutiful, obedient, and to live a strict Christian life. Caring for her younger siblings, doing chores at the house, and attending church took up most of her time outside of school.

Her desire to be a dutiful daughter was reflected in the expectations she had for me and my sisters. She was taught that if you loved and respected your parents, you would do what they say without question. But we were in Texas, far away from her island roots and the culture she knew. Her family was on the other side of the globe. She had expectations for what her family life would look like, and when those were out of reach, she struggled with her self-worth and hope for the future. The more uncertainty and stress, the greater her need to control the behavior of me and my siblings. Like so many other moms, she needed more support in raising her family and taking care of herself.

There was a long time where I wasn't aware I internalized my mom's bouts of unhappiness as an indication that I wasn't good enough to make her happy. It took becoming conscious not only of my LHBs but also the LHBs my parents grew up with to stop internalizing my childhood experiences as a personal failure. I came to realize, *Mom was really struggling with self-worth, and when you aren't conscious of your Higher Self, those fears of inadequacy easily get projected outward, even to your children.* My Higher Self empowered me to let go of resentment and see my mom for who she really is. She is not the sum of her mistakes, conditioning, trauma, or misgivings. She is her Higher Self, and that realization deepened my understanding and love for her.

Our Family Loves Us the Best Way They Know How

We never really stop wanting the approval, love, intimacy, nurturing, tenderness, compassion, quality time, and acceptance that we feel was missing in our childhoods—or in our family relationships now. And that is not easy.

But there is a difference between knowing these wounds are there and identifying with them. When you identify with them, you see yourself and the world through the fundamental belief that some part of you is lacking because something was missing from your childhood. You can never forgive, because your anger is helping to fill that void inside you. You will always see your family members and parent figures as the role they either fulfilled or didn't. And when you are with them, you will step into your role as a hurt child, as well.

Bringing your Higher Self to your familial relationships empowers you to be compassionate with your wounds while also understanding that this isn't the past and you are no longer a child who is dependent on the validation of others. You begin to respond differently to your triggers because you know triggers aren't who you are and therefore do not control you. You start getting in touch with what your actual needs and boundaries are in your familial relationships as an adult. You begin seeing your family members as individuals separate from your childhood story. Your parents and caregivers also grew up with a set of expectations, and if they didn't find a path to returning to their sense of wholeness and awakening to their essential natures — their Higher Selves — whatever belief of lack they carried with them got projected onto you. But it's not your responsibility to make them whole by becoming some version of yourself they want to see, never questioning their choices as parents, blaming yourself for their unhappiness, or hiding your authentic self.

Connecting to your Higher Self is the best way to honor where you came from and the experiences that you grew up with. In doing so, you alchemize the painful experiences into healing. You take part in ending the generational cycle of fear of inadequacy and set an example of self-love. Healing yourself is healing your family.

You can give yourself the love, nurturing, support, and compassion that you have always wanted. It's never too late. People assume they shouldn't need a certain type of encouragement, softness, or kindness just because they are no longer children. But those needs don't go away. We can take up the mantle and re-parent ourselves.

Chosen Family

There is nothing wrong with feeling a sense of responsibility to your family, caring about what they think, and wanting them to be proud of you. There is nothing wrong with wanting to be best friends with your siblings and to have picture-perfect relationships. But there is a difference between depending on that for your own self-worth and knowing you are worthy with or without fulfilling their desires or them fulfilling yours.

When you stand in the truth of your Higher Self, you can make choices that reflect your worth, keep healthy boundaries, continue healing your wounds, and redefine what family love really is. Family is more than biology or how we grew up; **family is interdependence with those who love and support you.** Today, I am so grateful for my chosen family: a group of very close friends who have been there for me through hard times and easy times. We have been in disagreements and misunderstandings, but we are committed to validating each other's needs and being on a path of inner growth together. I don't know how I would have gotten through the past ten years without them.

You can redefine what family means to you. You are not limited by the past. You can start your own traditions and rituals, create new boundaries, find new ways of showing and expressing love, and curate an emotionally safe and accepting home. Whether that is with biological family, romantic partners, friends, pets, or all of the above!

Last year, I adopted my first dog. And I have to say, I never thought I could love an animal so much! Rio is my baby, my child, and my family.

Compassion Isn't Condoning Behavior

Having compassion for your family doesn't mean that you are okay with all of their behaviors; it means you can see the truth behind those behaviors. It's possible to understand these behaviors as a product of a largely unhealed world—a world of injustice, shame, violence, racism, sexism, homophobia, and transphobia; a world that teaches that you must meet certain criteria to have value; a world where love, acceptance, and vulnerability are often viewed as weakness. In that context, it makes sense that one could be misguided in how one treats themselves and others. That doesn't mean you shouldn't require accountability, kindness, and compassion in your relationships; it means that if you have the capacity to change, unlearn, and heal, so do other people.

Healing the wounds

As my sisters and I grew older, both my parents changed a great deal. They became happier, healthier, and more joyous. They are extremely grateful to my older sister, Felili, for taking on so much responsibility in our younger years. A lot of these changes have to do with having much more financial stability and not having to be in fight-or-flight mode all the time. But it is also due to their own spiritual evolution. My mom and I have done so much healing in our relationship, have had difficult talks, cried, hugged, argued, and apologized. After I started creating the Higher Self memes, we began having more conversations about spirituality, God, love, and forgiveness. Moving beyond anger helped me begin receiving the softness and affection she now showers me with every time I see her.

Sometimes I wonder if I had grown up in my parents' generation, in their environment and circumstances, would I have made the same choices? Would I have been able to get through those challenging times the way they did? How would I have coped?

Often my family comes up in my meditation and prayer. And I consciously picture them smiling. It helps remind me of their true spirits, the love that radiates within them, and how much they deserve peace, acceptance, and healing — just like me. It helps me remember that we are actually healing each other.

"It was really hard to grow up, because I wanted to do all the fun things, but I couldn't."

My mom told me this over the phone from her suburban house in Dallas, while I sat at my desk in my office in upstate New York, drawing doodles of hearts and eyes on my notebook like I used to do as a kid. Outside my office window, snow had begun to fall, and I thought about how lucky I was to get to live in New York and experience it, like I'd fantasized about in Texas as a child whenever I'd watch Christmas movies. Before I started writing this book, I knew I wanted to ask my mom questions about how she grew up. Aside from the occasional story here and there, she rarely talked about her upbringing with me and my sisters.

"Like, what fun things couldn't you do as a kid?" I asked her.

"Sometimes we wanted to go outside and play but we couldn't. I had that too like my parents, the need to feel in control as a mother, you know, that idea of being afraid something is going to happen to my kids if I let them go. Not realizing that you have to let your children go to experience things, and they will learn."

After the phone call with my mom, I packed up for the day and headed to the parking lot. Everything was covered in a thick layer of bright white: the cars, the sidewalks, the restaurant across the street — snow overtaking everything, seeming to stop time. I stood still for a moment and watched the individual snowflakes, each particle floating down slowly, landing ever so gently on top of each other. I thought about how all the thin layers of snow build up to turn into something so heavy, so powerful, and how I was the embodiment of all the layers of experiences in my lineage — all the hardships and the triumphs. I caught a few flakes and watched them melt away on the warmth of my hands, which, with every passing year, remind me more of my mother's.

You Are So Lovable

You have always been enough just for being you. You are born whole, and deserving of tenderness, acceptance, and compassion. You are part of all creation, connected to every living being through an interconnected web of divine consciousness. Healing isn't about changing or trying to fix parts of yourself—it's about returning to who you have always been.

Our family relationships aren't easy to navigate, and healing our childhood wounds isn't simple, but being grounded in your Higher Self empowers you to realize you are worth it.

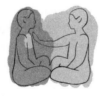

Harnessing Your Higher Self When Addressing Family Relationships and Childhood

1. **Stop shaming yourself for your family struggles.** Can we all just agree to stop internalizing the dysfunction in our family as some kind of personal failure or inadequacy? Family dysfunction is a product of a world that doesn't teach us our worth or how to authentically love one another. It's hard enough to process our childhoods; you don't need to add

another layer of pain on top of that. There is nothing wrong with you.

2. **Set boundaries.** It's very common to grow up in a family household where boundaries were basically nonexistent. Where parents read your diary or searched your room. Where you weren't allowed to shut your door. Where parental figures put you in emotionally unsafe situations by forcing you to spend time with people that you didn't like or made you uncomfortable. Or maybe guilted you into performing for their guests when they came over (me) and now it feels nearly impossible to say no when your mom asks you to Sunday dinner.

    When you set boundaries, it may upset some family members, but it is the first step to a healthy and autonomous relationship. Otherwise, resentment can lead to anger until the relationship is no longer authentic. Boundaries are often a very new concept for family members. So, set an example! Teach them something new! If you are ever unsure whether doing something with family violates your boundaries or is emotionally safe, ask yourself if you are able to embody your Higher Self in that environment. Is it a place or experience where you feel safe to be yourself, to love yourself, and accept yourself? I don't mean an environment where you are confident everyone sees you and accepts your authenticity (although that would definitely be ideal)—but is their energy keeping you from staying grounded in your own self-worth? At different times in our healing journey, different environments/relationships can be helpful, tolerable, or more harmful and possibly retraumatizing. It's good to keep in mind that your boundaries can change, so if something that used to feel comfortable no longer does, it might be time to reassess.

3. **Be proud of yourself for ending the cycle of harm.** Every time you acknowledge how worthy you are of love and care and abundance, you are helping to end a cycle of wounds

perpetuated by unaddressed trauma and dysfunction. Every time you choose to unlearn the LHBs you picked up in your childhood home, you are resonating as a force of acceptance and love that is so needed in your lineage. Every time you show up to therapy or to work on yourself through other healing modalities, you are giving yourself the time, love, and attention you need so you don't repeat the cycles of harm from your upbringing. You are very courageous.

4. **Stop believing you can control your family members' choices.** Wouldn't it be great if your parental figures and/or caregivers would become what you have always wanted them to be? Wouldn't it be great to get that apology you always wanted, or for their politics to align with yours? Wouldn't it be great if your sibling didn't cause so much strife in your family or argue with you at Thanksgiving? Wouldn't it be great if your uncle wasn't transphobic and didn't forbid your nephew from dressing up like a Disney princess on Halloween? The more we try to control our family members, the more disappointed we will be. If we want to be a force for healing and change in our families, the best way is to lead by example. Live your life authentically, with accountability, compassion, and healthy boundaries. Stay on your healing path. Rather than needing them to change so you can be happy, change what you need from them.

5. **If you are trying to process trauma from your childhood, you need to seek guidance and support from those with experience and expertise.** Therapy should be free for everyone. Unfortunately, that is not the case. If you have insurance or are able to pay for a therapist, please prioritize doing so. There are also many places that offer sliding scale prices (especially for LGBTQ+ identified folks) or cheaper group therapies. Beyond therapy, there is support available. One of the benefits of the internet is easier access to the work of licensed therapists and psychologists. There are many books that are great resources on trauma and online healing groups accessible to all.

I've learned a lot from therapists I follow on social media. I've put some recommendations in the Further Reading section of this book. Do some research. Ask around. Help is out there.

6. **Understand that you are not unlovable because someone important in your life didn't know how to love you. That was their limitation, not yours. Let go of that story.** Being mistreated, abused, neglected, or put down by the people who are supposed to love and protect you is heartbreaking. No one deserves that. Sometimes we can clearly trace the cyclical nature of the harmful behavior in our families, like generations of physical or sexual abuse, untreated mental illness, or a family history of alcoholism or drug abuse. Or sometimes this turmoil seems to appear out of nowhere. For no "logical" reason. Either way, no matter the cause, what we experience are the effects—the pain, the sorrow, the loss, the fear, the anger. But remember: You are no longer a scared child unable to care for, protect, or defend yourself. You are free. You are on the path of healing. Nothing that anyone ever did to you can diminish your spirit, your light, and your capacity to love and be loved. You are so lovable.

LHBs About Family and Childhood vs. Higher Self

LHB: Having childhood trauma means there will always be something wrong with me.

Higher Self: Going through traumatic experiences does not mean there is anything wrong with you; it means you were in a circumstance beyond your control and you deserve all the care and support to keep healing those wounds.

LHB: It's too late to address my childhood.

Higher Self: There is no right or wrong time to be ready to address your wounds. Whenever you feel called, that is the right time for you.

LHB: In order to heal I need the person who hurt me to acknowledge what they did.

Higher Self: In order to heal, you need to stop believing the person who hurt you can heal you.

LHB: You can't say no to a relationship with a family member if you unconditionally love them.

Higher Self: Unconditional love does not mean unconditionally putting up with harmful relationships. Often, the loving thing to do is walk away.

Affirmations

* I am not my wounds.
* I don't have to let go of my past—my past was an experience. I just have to let go of the belief that those experiences define me.
* My family loves me the best way they know how.
* I have always been lovable.
* I can give myself the nurturing, kindness, and compassion I have always wanted from my family.
* The best way to honor my past is to be an example of love.

Writing Exercise: Love Letter to Your Younger Self

For this exercise you will need a childhood photo. It can be on your phone. If you don't have access to a childhood photo, you can look up an image that reminds you of childhood, perhaps from your favorite cartoon, or you can use an object of sentimental value, like your old teddy bear.

Take out the photo, image, or object and in your journal or on a piece of paper write your younger self a letter. Write all the loving, compassionate, and nurturing things that would have been so helpful to hear at that age. Tell your younger self how lovable they have always been. Tell your younger self to keep your head up. There is no right way to write this letter. Let your heart guide you.

Meditation for Family Healing

Pick a quiet place where you will not be interrupted. It might be helpful to put on some peaceful meditation music, or you can sit in silence. Close your eyes and slowly begin to focus on your breath, until you feel your whole body begin to relax. Visualize a bright light radiating from your heart. Imagine that white, warm light spreading all over your body. Until you feel like you are glowing. The warm white light is your connection to your Higher Self—your inner radiating love . . .

Relax and breathe. Without opening your eyes, visualize someone in your family sitting across from you. Whoever comes to mind first. Picture them smiling, peaceful. Stay there for a moment until you feel a calm presence from them. Now imagine sending your warm bright light from your heart to theirs. Radiate that light from your heart space to light up their heart space. This is your Higher Self connecting to theirs. To their inner essence. Not their behavior or personality or mistakes—their spirit, where the two of you are connected in a higher dimension of conscious, loving awareness.

Sit with this connection until you intuitively know when to stop. End the meditation with a mantra: "I honor the love in you. I honor the love within myself."

Journal Prompts

1. Thoughts and/or feelings of inadequacy that I carry from my childhood are...

2. Flip the script: My Higher Self would respond to those thoughts by saying...

3. Ways I can give myself more grace and compassion when it comes to my childhood wounds are...

4. If I could guess what LHBs that my parental figures/caregivers carried with them while I was growing up they would be...

5. Ways that those LHBs affected me are...

6. Behavior changes (if any) that I can make to have better boundaries with my family are...

7. I am lovable because...

8. My definition of family is...

Chapter 6

Dating

Me: *I'm looking for that one person out there who will complete me.*
Higher Self: *I'm right here!!!!*

Swipe life

After a bad breakup in 2015, I downloaded my first dating app. At first, it was exciting. All of a sudden, there were so many faces to choose from, so much possibility. It felt as though finding a good match was inevitable. But a few months in, the thrill of swiping through countless profiles and photos was replaced by frustration and boredom. Sitting in my apartment, I'd lie in the same position in bed, scrolling my phone for so long that my thumb would get numb. Still, I couldn't stop. I felt like those people I'd seen at casinos in Atlantic City in velour sweatsuits, cigarettes hanging out of their mouths, spending hours on the slot machines, convincing themselves that this was the day they were gonna hit the jackpot.

I'd spend less than a second looking at each profile picture, trying to maximize the efficiency of my swipes. Tyra, 32, *nope*...Lizzy, 28, *nah*...Jackie, 29, *maybe?*...I'd scroll through a few more of Jackie, 29's photos and see one of her hugging an Elmo doll. *Ummm, no, definitely not.* Sam, 35...*yes*...ding ding ding! It's a match!

Dating Culture

Our contemporary concept of dating—two people going out together in a public setting—was not part of American culture until the late 1800s/early 1900s. Industrialization provided more independence from family expectations and changed how people made and spent money. Restaurants, dance halls, and theaters had become more commonplace, and colleges and workplaces provided more opportunity for people to meet. Dating was no longer just a precursor to marriage—it had become an opportunity to socialize.

Whether you are dating to find a potential partner for marriage, or just looking for a casual hookup, one thing we don't often think about is how the culture we are raised in and the Learned Hierarchical Beliefs of our society influence our dating experiences—sometimes, in ways that are detrimental to our well-being, self-acceptance, and joy.

According to our culture's LHBs, you need to look a certain way, accomplish certain things, and have certain possessions in order to be desirable. Your perceived value will determine how "datable" you are. Dating culture has long been a place where sexism, racial bias, classism, fatphobia, heteronormative bias, and ableism have run rampant.

This messaging is reinforced by popular culture. Just look at movies and TV—the "datable" love interests are mostly cis, thin, white passing, able-bodied, neurotypical, and straight.

Our Learned Hierarchical Beliefs around romantic desirability are also conditioned by our familial upbringing. Parent figures and family members may have pushed you to look and behave a certain way in order to fit into their idea of what is attractive and desirable. They probably also had ideas about the desirable and attractive qualities you should seek in a potential mate.

You may have been raised to believe you shouldn't date anyone of a different race, class, or religion, or anyone who wasn't straight or cis. Or your guardians may have tried to find your mate for you—putting their preferences ahead of yours.

If you are not conscious of your own LHBs, you will not be able to distinguish what qualities in a person are important to your Higher Self from the qualities that matter according to the biases you were conditioned to believe in. You will also judge your own value according to your LHBs. This not only puts pressure on every date to either make or break your confidence, but it also takes away the humanity of the experience, because people are merely reflections of where you stand in the hierarchy of the dating pool.

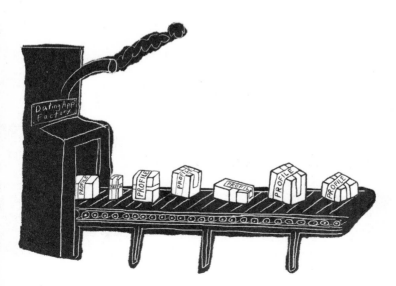

Sam, 35

On the night of my date with Sam, 35, I had a couple of drinks at a bar before getting in a cab to meet them. This was my normal routine prior to meeting up with someone from a dating app—partaking of some "liquid courage." You'd think I wouldn't have been so anxious, especially because since my last breakup, I had gone on as many dates as possible. It was the only thing that distracted me from feeling lonely or having to confront the difficult emotions left over from my relationship ending. I wasn't looking for anything serious, and most of my dates were either total disappointments or, on the more successful end of the spectrum, drunk hookups, which at the time felt like exactly what I needed.

In the Uber from the bar, I took out my phone to look at Sam, 35's profile again. There was only one picture, them posing with their dog. I thought it was a bold move to only supply *one* picture, and to have it be with their dog, but I let it slide. Their bio said they were a graphic designer (which could mean anything from designing Oscar-winning film posters to brunch menus); they enjoyed rock climbing, liked to cook (bonus), and had recently moved to New York from the West Coast (also a bonus, because that minimized the chance we had slept with the same people—sometimes the queer scene in New York feels very small).

The cab pulled up to Trophy Bar on Broadway, and I took a deep breath to psych myself up. There was only one person sitting by themselves at the bar. It was Sam, 35, and I was immediately disappointed. They didn't look as attractive as their profile picture—as if they took that picture years ago on a really, really good day. I took a quick scan of their outfit—pretty basic, something they probably bought at Old Navy or an outdoorsy-type store that also sells hiking boots.

Oh God, are those Crocs? The lack of enthusiasm was audible in my voice as I approached them.

"Hi, Sam?"

Sam looked up with a friendly smile. "Hi, Bunny."

After small talk about where we were both coming from, and what we did that day, I was desperate to order a drink. When you decide you are not interested in hooking up with your date, it's best not to seem too friendly. So I wasn't giving Sam, 35, a lot of eye contact. When the bartender finally approached, I ordered a tequila soda and Sam ordered a...Diet Coke.

Oh my God, what? I thought to myself.

"I don't drink alcohol," Sam said when they noticed my confused facial expression.

"Oh, that's cool," I said.

Wow, this is really not going to be fun.

After about forty-five minutes of awkward conversation, during which I showed the bare minimum of interest, I told Sam, 35, I needed to go home to feed my cat. The date was a total disappointment, and I couldn't wait to go home, eat some ramen noodles, and forget all about it.

They also got up to leave, which didn't surprise me, because why would you stay at a bar by yourself drinking Diet Cokes?

"Where do you live, maybe we can share an Uber?" Sam, 35, asked.

I hesitated at first, worried they would take it as a signal I didn't want the date to be over. But I changed my mind when I thought about how much money I'd spent the last couple of months on Ubers.

"I live on MacDonough and Saratoga."

"Wait, that's where I live!"

Yeah, right.

"Oh, okay," I said, sarcastically.

"No, really, I live at Seven Thirty-Five MacDonough."

Oh my God. That is two doors down from me. So much for me forgetting about this date. Sam, 35, is my freakin' neighbor.

Connecting to my Higher Self helped me reflect back on this time period and realize my unconscious LHBs had kept me in a constant state of fear of my own inadequacy; therefore, projecting inadequacy on other people was how I self-soothed. *At least I am better than this person.* But I was not better than Sam, 35. They were friendly, intelligent, and mature. They were my neighbor, and could have been a friend, if I'd acknowledged them as a person rather than just a "bad Tinder date." I cringe thinking about how rude I must have seemed and how I assumed they weren't any fun because they were sober, especially knowing how difficult it is to be sober when you are going on dates with people you don't know. It takes real confidence in your choices. A confidence that I didn't have back then. I was struggling with my drinking at the time, numbing my feelings of rejection from my breakup with alcohol. But rather than realizing Sam's Diet Coke was triggering my own issues, I projected my discomfort onto them as a character flaw.

I also looked down on them for what they were wearing, which is especially ironic now that I wear Crocs *all the time*. Since I was also using hookups to gain my confidence, when I decided I wasn't physically attracted enough to hook up with them, the whole evening became a waste of my time. If I met Sam, 35 now, they would be someone I would want to hang out with. Because now I understand how my own biases and fears of inadequacy can make me believe perfectly lovely people aren't worthy of my time and attention.

Apps Make It Easy—But Not in the Way You Thought

The convenience and efficiency of dating apps—being able to scroll through countless dating profiles at once, making snap judgments based on a handful of photographs and a few bits of information—make it easier to objectify potential romantic connections according to your Learned Hierarchical Beliefs, and harder to see the humanity in people and in yourself. Every potential connection becomes a product advertised online. A product that either meets your standards on the ladder of "desirable" qualities or not. And you also begin to see *yourself* as a product, judging your value based on how many people want to put in an order for you. If you believe a person's value is based on how much money they make, you will dismiss anyone who has a low-paying job. If you believe a person's value is based on the shape of their body, you will never try to get to know someone if they wear a certain dress size. Why? Because if they aren't good enough from the lens of your LHBs, they won't ever be able to make *you* feel good enough. Dating apps are not in themselves responsible for creating your Learned Hierarchical Beliefs, but similar to social media, they can exacerbate them.

From the Higher Self perspective, every person has value, and no one is better than anyone else. And in order to make authentic connections and have meaningful experiences, we need to become more aware of the biases that we bring to our dating life, about ourselves and other people. We need to question our assumptions.

We are all in the process of unlearning our racist, fatphobic, classist, ableist, and patriarchal conditioning. To pretend those Learned Hierarchical Beliefs do not color our opinions about potential mates and our opinions about our own value is to be in denial.

I'm not saying you are supposed to be attracted to every person you meet or expect every person to be attracted to you. I'm saying we all should take a deeper look into why we find certain qualities attractive and why we assume certain qualities about ourselves are unattractive. Are you dating with the wisdom of your Higher Self—that knows you are no better than anyone else and no one is better than you—or are your Learned Hierarchical Beliefs having you chase validation by using dating as a means to enforce the delusion of your inadequacy? Because that is what the lens of our LHBs wants you to believe—that you aren't inherently valuable just for being you, that you need to keep finding outside validation in order to be enough, and that you need to do whatever is necessary to keep climbing that hierarchical social ladder.

He pretended I no longer existed.

Ezra was a senior in my high school when I was a sophomore. He was popular, tall, and funny. I never thought he had noticed me until one day he came up and asked for my number. I was surprised. I was a sophomore, and a popular senior was asking for my number. Excited, I gave it to him.

Later that night I was watching a rerun of *My So-Called Life,* the episode when Angela thought Jordan Catalano's song he wrote about his car was about her, when the phone rang. It was Ezra calling to ask me to go with him to senior prom. Of course I said yes.

I remember the look on his face when he picked me up on prom night and I told him my curfew was eleven thirty. He was disappointed. Little did he know I had to fight tooth and nail with my mom to even go to prom and be able to stay out that late. But his disappointment didn't get me down; I was excited to be wearing my new yellow dress I got at Dillard's, to get my first flower corsage, and to be one of the only sophomores at prom.

We spent most of the date hanging out with his friends in the parking lot outside the dance, while they smoked joints, joked around, and made out with their dates. I barely said a word. Every now and then, Ezra would ask a few "getting to know you" questions. He was polite, and before he dropped me off, we kissed for a while in his car until I said I had to go in.

The following week, Ezra asked if I wanted to hang out after school. I hadn't felt we had much of a connection, but I felt guilty for not being able to stay out all night on our prom date, like he had missed out by choosing me. I thought we would go out to eat or to a movie, but he said we should just hang out at his house.

He took me straight to his bedroom. We started making out on his black and white plaid comforter, and after a little bit, he got up and went into the bathroom and came out carrying a condom. It wasn't the first time I'd had sex—I had lost my virginity in the eighth grade. And even though I really would have preferred to talk and get to know each other more first, I did it anyway. He was older and had much more social status than me at our school. I thought I was lucky he liked me, and I wanted to let him know I liked him too. Were we boyfriend and girlfriend now?

Ezra didn't ask me on any more dates after that, no more phone calls, no more smiles in the hallway, no explanation. It was like it never happened. *What did I do wrong?* I wondered. *Did he not like my body? Did I say something stupid? Was I not cool enough?*

The rejection made me feel like not only was I not good enough for Ezra to want to date again, but that I was so insignificant, no explanation was warranted. I was rendered invisible.

Ghosting vs. Setting Boundaries

Ghosting, the act of cutting off all communication with someone without any explanation, is becoming more common in dating culture than ever. According to a 2018 academic study, 25.3 percent of people have been ghosted by a romantic partner and 21.7 percent have ghosted other people. When it comes to dating, ghosting is often seen as totally acceptable behavior, especially when the connection was made online. Just as technology has made it more convenient to scroll through countless potential romantic connections, it has also made it easier to disappear.

There are many theories about why people ghost: fear of confrontation, lack of empathy, feeling overwhelmed, not wanting to hurt someone's feelings, trying to avoid rejection, and even narcissism.

No matter the reason, ghosting says more about the person doing the ghosting than the person who is ghosted. Yet when we are ghosted, we feel hurt, confused, and disposable. It can feel especially cruel after physical intimacy.

From the Higher Self perspective, everyone's needs are valid because everyone is valuable. Needing to end things with another person, or not being interested in them romantically, is not a testament to them not being good enough for you. If you think someone isn't good enough for you, then of course it's easy to feel guilty for telling them you're not interested anymore. Maybe it's easier to just ignore that person. Deep down, though, the underlying belief is that you think they aren't on your level according to the hierarchy of worth you were conditioned to believe in.

Similarly, if you see yourself through that hierarchical lens, if someone isn't interested in you or no longer wants to date you, you will internalize that as you not being good enough for them. And you interpret a communication of "I'm not interested" as "You are not worthy of hanging out with me." It also brings to the surface other LHBs like feeling inadequately attractive or feeling socially inferior, as was the case with my first ghosting in high school. This delusional lens is common, and makes dating a game of winners and losers. And it makes sense that in a game where people are just trying to win a higher spot on the ladder of self-worth, ghosting someone confirms the belief that the ghoster is superior to the ghosted.

Don't get me wrong—sometimes it is necessary to cut off contact. Especially when it comes to your safety. If someone has crossed your boundaries, it's safe to assume that communicating another boundary—that you don't want to see them anymore—will be futile or even dangerous. And you shouldn't have to put yourself in that position. But there is a difference between setting a boundary and ghosting. Ghosting is when you are unwilling to communicate your boundaries—which is really about being accountable to your own feelings, needs, and desires. On the contrary, cutting off contact because your boundaries have been violated is being accountable to yourself—showing yourself that you don't need to feel unsafe with that person again.

In a culture where we are not used to setting boundaries, particularly those who are socialized as female and made to feel like their needs are less valid, setting them in dating can feel uncomfortable. But there is nothing wrong with respecting your needs. Here are some examples of go-to words and phrases when setting boundaries in dating.

"No."

"I'm not into that."

"I'm not interested in an exclusive partnership."

"I don't want to do that."

"I don't want to go on a date with you."

"I don't think we are compatible."

"This is not working out for me."

These might seem kind of obvious, but many of us feel like they are not okay to say. They absolutely are! Being honest is way more kind than disappearing and/or pretending someone doesn't exist.

Some people believe any form of ghosting is not okay, including not responding after a few DMs have been exchanged. Some people think ghosting is not acceptable after a certain number of dates. I'm not here to tell you where to draw the line. But having clear boundaries with people you are dating and communicating your intentions and needs, even when it's not convenient, isn't just a more empathetic and humane way to treat another person;

it is a practice in self-acceptance. When you are open with others about your needs—by telling them the level of commitment you are interested in, and/or being honest when the relationship is no longer something you feel aligned with—you are also sending yourself a message that your needs, desires, and intentions are valid enough to be communicated.

Trust the Timing

What if you feel like you aren't finding any success in dating? Keep in mind that the seemingly endless pool of potential dates in the apps creates an illusion that you should find lots of success, and if you are not, there must be something wrong with you. However, research suggests that having more options does not equate to finding more successful matches.

Then there is the messaging by popular culture you grew up with and are still bombarded by today: family members who are always asking about your love life, or the pressure to bring a date to a social event, like a New Year's Eve party. Your Higher Self knows that these dynamics are not a reflection of your true self, and you don't have to buy into them. You are whole just how you are, and remembering that will enable you to trust that the romantic connection you are looking for will happen when the timing is right.

Self-worth should not depend on the status of your dating life, whether you are looking for a casual hookup or dating to find a potential long-term partnership. We are all on the journey of unlearning our LHBs and connecting to the place where our true validation lies—within us. And the sooner you realize that, the greater your chance of finding a romantic connection in the future that is a reflection of what you deserve.

When you acknowledge that your LHBs influence how you see yourself and others in the dating world, you can start to build more awareness of your self-worth, intentions, boundaries, and expectations when it comes to dating. When you bring the consciousness of your Higher Self with you, you are aware that you deserve honesty, compassion, respect, and accountability. Both for yourself and for other people. You are honest about the type of relationship you are looking for, you are aware of what your boundaries are when it comes to physical intimacy, and you are unashamed of your needs and desires. You are also aware that everyone you meet is also conditioned by their own LHBs and fears of inadequacy.

There will be people along the way who are misguided. There will be people who think that mistreating someone else makes them powerful. There will be people who project their insecurities onto you. But you will know that has nothing to do with how worthy you are. You will know that true power doesn't come from making someone feel inadequate. It comes from the realization that you are enough, and you always have been. Dating is not a game with winners and losers. It's an opportunity to have an authentic experience and to allow your Higher Self to guide you to the relationships that will support you on your journey of self-acceptance.

You deserve respect and honesty from all your dating experiences. You are a joy to be around. You have always been enough. Wherever your dating life takes you, bring that truth with you.

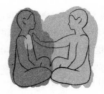

Bring Your Higher Self to Dating

1. **Investigate your LHBs.** What assumptions are you making about people and where do those come from? What ways are you unkind to yourself, and who put that thought into your head? Becoming aware of your LHBs is the first step to disempowering them.

2. **Give yourself compassion and patience when LHBs come to the surface.** Some days are going to be easier than others. If you find yourself in a spiral of insecurity, rather than adding another layer of self-criticism for being insecure, give yourself grace and send yourself some love. We all get tender. We are human. Your Higher Self wants you to know that no matter what you're going through, you are enough.

3. **Keep in mind that the person on the other side of the screen you are swiping on is a human being with feelings, opinions, fears, LHBs, insecurities, desires, and dreams.** Dating apps and social media have made it so easy to dehumanize the person behind the digital avatar you are interacting with. But dehumanizing them not only keeps you from a perspective of compassion and mutual respect; it also makes you vulnerable to forgetting that if someone is unkind, disrespectful, or inappropriate, it's because of their unhealed issues. Not because there is something wrong with you.

4. **Just because the date didn't work out doesn't mean it was a failure.** Sometimes we get so caught up in finding the "right" person for us that if a date doesn't "measure up" or check

the right boxes, the entire experience becomes a failure or a waste of time. Or if someone isn't interested in us, we feel like we failed. But dating is not a test of your value. Stop grading yourself.

Your Higher Self uses every experience as an opportunity to see yourself and the world through the lens of love. If you ever feel disheartened after a date that wasn't the right connection, ask yourself, *How can I give myself love right now?*

5. **Trust the red flags.** We've all been on a date where the other person seemed uninterested, or showed up late without apologizing, or said something offensive, or made a disparaging comment about a server. But we really want things to work out, so we question whether we are being too judgmental or if we should trust this feeling of unease. If you are feeling bad on a date or someone is rubbing you the wrong way, you don't need proof that there is something wrong with that person—you can simply acknowledge that you are not compatible and leave it there. There is a difference between feeling nervous around someone new and feeling bad around them. Trust what your heart is telling you.

6. **Never meet up or talk with someone if any part of you intuitively feels unsafe.** Our Higher Selves are like compasses guiding us to the awareness of our worth. But listening to that guidance isn't always easy. Especially if you're not used to trusting yourself. A lot of people engage in risky dating behavior because they really want to meet someone, need an ego boost, or really want to have a fun hookup despite their better judgment. Feeling lonely or being horny is never worth putting your physical and emotional well-being at risk. Your life is sacred. Take care of yourself!

Affirmations

Pro tip: These are especially great to say before you leave your home to go on a date.

- I trust in the divine timing of my life and am open to all possibilities.
- My most important goals are self-acceptance, compassion, and inner peace.
- I see the humanity in all people.
- I am worthy of kindness, respect, and joyful experiences.
- My relationship status does not determine my worth.
- Being single is an opportunity to know myself more deeply. I honor this time.

Writing Exercise

Step 1

Make a list of the qualities you find important in someone you are dating and put them into two categories: important to your LHBs and important to your Higher Self. Remember: LHBs are the lens of social hierarchy and cultural bias (seeing something as good or bad in comparison to others); Higher Self is seeing qualities through the lens of the inherent worth and value of all human beings. Don't worry about seeming superficial. No one is going to see this list but you, so be honest. For example, maybe an important quality in someone you date is being over five-seven. Put that in the LHB category, because it's about finding taller people more attractive. Another example is that you are attracted to people who are kind to you—that goes into the Higher Self category, because it reflects your inherent value. Again, putting qualities in the LHB category does not mean they are bad or that you are a superficial jerk—we are just creating awareness around the motivation for your preferences.

Step 2

Make the same list about qualities you feel other people in the dating world would find attractive or unattractive about you. Divide those qualities in two categories—LHBs and Higher Self qualities. Don't worry about seeming vain or superficial. No one is going to see this but you, so be honest. If one thing on your list is "I am prettier than most people," put that in the LHB category. If it's "I'm beautiful inside and out," put that in the Higher Self category. If one quality is "I don't make enough money for a thirty-year-old," put that in LHB. If it's "I am working on knowing I deserve abundance just like everyone else," put that in Higher Self. Remember: There is no right or wrong here. Two people might be talking about the same characteristic but see it from different perspectives.

Step 3

Look over each list carefully. Go through the LHB side of each list and journal about some of the possible reasons you think you have those preferences for dating partners, or those beliefs about yourself and your qualities. Could it be you feel insecure about your body because popular culture has told you your body doesn't fit into a certain beauty standard? Could you want to find someone who has a six-figure salary because your mom told you a good partner is one with a lot of money? Again, this isn't about being self-critical or even changing any of your opinions. It's about taking time to bring more awareness to why you have those opinions and expectations.

Step 4

Now that you have spent some time thinking and journaling about your preferences, beliefs, and which qualities are important to you when dating other people (and what qualities about yourself you feel you have to offer), see if any qualities you have in the LHB section can be seen through the lens of your Higher Self or eliminated from the LHB section completely. For example, if you put "I'm not cool enough" in the LHB section of personal characteristics, and realized that part of the reason you feel that way is because you were bullied by some jerks in middle school, and you've been holding on to the words of a few thirteen-year-olds for years, you can rewrite it as "I'm unlearning the belief that I'm not cool enough" and put it in the Higher Self qualities. Or, if you realized that your preference for dating only cis males has more to do with fear of judgment than your actual interests, you can erase that preference completely.

NOTE: This list can be ongoing, updated, and something that you return to if you ever feel bogged down with self-judgment and insecurity while dating. It is also a good reminder to keep your heart and mind open to possibility when looking for or meeting someone new, or if you feel you might have some walls you want to work on letting go of. You can work on Higher Selfing your preferences and learned beliefs about dating at any point in time.

Journal Prompts

1. LHBs that I bring to my dating life are . . .

    _____

2. Past experiences and/or influences that put those beliefs in my head are . . .

    _____

3. Flip the script: My Higher Self would respond to my LHBs by telling me . . .

    _____

4. Some changes in behavior and/or boundaries that will better serve me when it comes to dating are...

_____

5. I am amazing because...

_____

Chapter 7

Committed Relationships

Me: *Why are relationships so hard?*
Higher Self: *Your partner triggers the part of you that most needs to be healed, and you trigger the part of your partner that most needs to be healed, and that is no accident. It's why you met.*

Finding "the one" scared the crap out of me.

Two weeks after I got married, I sent my spouse, Khara, a text.

I'm going to shave my head.

That morning, I'd awakened with a powerful urge to change my appearance. Normally when I had that feeling, I just changed my hair color. I've dyed it pink, blue, green, orange, red — pretty much every color you can think of — since I was a teenager. Hair shows the passing of time; I treated mine like a scrapbook of split ends and Manic Panic.

But that day, I needed to do something more drastic.

In preparation for my wedding, I spent eight months growing my hair long. I felt pressure to look like the image of the beautiful brides I saw growing up in movies and on TV and magazine covers, with flowing locks and a facial expression that says, "This is the happiest day of my life." I can't tell you how many times I heard that on your wedding day, you are supposed to feel the most beautiful you have ever felt. Dang, that is a lot of pressure!

Two hours later, I was in the barber's chair at a queer-owned hair salon in Park Slope, watching my long bleached-blond locks fall to the ground, forming a pile on the floor, the buzz of the clippers zoning me out like a salon version of a white noise machine.

"All done!" said my giddy hairdresser, incredibly stoked to assist in my transformation.

I looked in the mirror and saw myself sans hair, and it hit me: The bride stage was officially over. The new stage of my life...marriage, was just beginning.

I made it. I found the person I am going to spend the rest of my life with. I finally settled down. I should feel at ease. I should feel...complete. Instead I was full of anxiety.

I assumed getting married would give me confidence, turn me into this secure person, because I finally had proof that I was lovable. Someone chose me! But I didn't feel any different. I was still insecure. I was still unsure of myself. Khara and I still had the same problems we had before the wedding. Getting married wasn't a magic fix for my issues or the relationship's, and I was terrified.

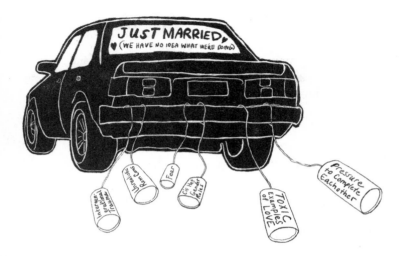

And They Lived Happily Ever After

It's not a coincidence that most movies about love and romance end with a wedding celebration: the happy couple, who almost didn't make it, share a kiss at the altar. That is where the story ends, because once you are married, everything will be okay. We all know relationships don't work that way. But movie producers don't think audiences want to see a story about trying to make a long-term relationship work. There's nothing glamorous about bickering, financial ups and downs, setting boundaries, learning about each other's wounds, and sharing responsibilities. Watching a couple discover new ways to communicate about who is going to do the dishes doesn't exactly scream, "I was on the edge of my seat!"

What popular culture did teach us was that getting married legitimizes love in a partnership. And that once you cross the altar you are complete.

Marriage Does Not Legitimize Love

We were taught that marriage is the pinnacle of true love. But for millennia, marriage had little to do with love. In her book *Marriage, a History,* Stephanie Coontz illustrates that what is often referred to in contemporary times as a "traditional" marriage is not as traditional as we think. People have always fallen in love, but love and the institution of marriage historically had little to do with one another. Throughout history in cultures all over the world, marriage has been a means to secure political and economic stability within a society, and a transaction to consolidate wealth and property. Since ancient times, married women were commonly viewed as the property of their husbands, expected to submit to their will and authority.

According to Coontz, the onset of the Enlightenment and the freedoms of the market economy in western Europe brought radical shifts to the social role of marriage. By the end of the 1700s, most marriages were based on personal choice rather than solely on economic stability.

Still, marrying for personal choice and not just economic security did not obliterate classist, patriarchal, and religiously oppressive LHBs from continuing to establish the cultural expectations of marriage. For centuries the role of a wife was to stay home and care for the children while the husband was the sole breadwinner. Despite gender roles being increasingly more fluid today, only 16 percent of households in the United States have the wife as the singular income earner.

Marriage is seen as the moral high ground by both religious doctrine and culture standards. Having a child "out of wedlock" could bring stigma and shame to individuals and families. Young people who get pregnant are often pressured to get married because it is the "right thing to do," even though it very often isn't. Unmarried and/or single parents are more often judged as not being fully capable of caring for their children than married couples are, regardless of the fact that marriage is not an antidote to abuse, neglect, and toxic behavior in families.

The institution of marriage has also not been immune to the insidiousness of racism, homophobia, and transphobia in our culture.

It wasn't until 1967 that the Supreme Court case of *Loving v. Virginia* finally granted legal protection for interracial marriages in the United States. Same-sex marriage became legal in all fifty states in the U.S. in 2015, but is still banned in most countries around the world. Today, trans people face marriage discrimination in the U.S. because not all state or local officials provide a marriage license that reflects their gender identity.

Sanctioned by social, political, and religious authority, marriage was to establish a social, moral, and political ideal within a society. That ideal has been shaped by a history of patriarchy, classism, racism, homophobia, and transphobia.

Marriage is so ingrained as the standard in society that many of us have never questioned why we want to get married. *Is this something that I really want, or was I just taught that in order to be happy and successful in life I needed to get married?* The LHB that marriage (particularly that between a man and a woman) is a higher form of love and commitment perpetuates the narrative that you must take part in this institution to have a sustainable and loving partnership, which is not the case. It also maintains that marriage can be a solution for your fears of inadequacy and/or a relationship that is struggling, because once you are married the relationship will be secure — and so will you. But marriage cannot fix those problems.

How We Learned to Love

In addition to the narratives of popular culture and society's hierarchical views on marriage, the examples of love we grew up with in our home greatly influence our beliefs about romantic partnership. We learned from watching how our parental figures treated each other, and how they communicated, shared responsibility, and displayed affection. We witnessed cultural traditions and gender roles play out in the home. Many of us watched the disillusionment of our parents' marriage and/or experienced the absence of a parent. Many of us sadly witnessed toxic behavior, turmoil, and domestic abuse.

It isn't just the way the adults in our life treated each other that taught us about love, but how they treated *us*. Our caregivers' level of affection toward us—their consistency, acceptance, love, and attention—fed us a narrative about how much love, attention, consistency, and acceptance we deserved. And we bring those beliefs with us as we grow older.

Attachment theory, a psychological and evolutionary theory developed by the psychiatrist John Bowlby, says attachments we form as early as infancy have lasting effects on the attachments we form into adulthood. According to him, "We do as we are done by."

If you had difficulties feeling loved by your caregivers, those experiences can form LHBs that you don't deserve to be loved in your adult relationships. If you were mistreated by a caregiver who was supposed to love you, you can mistake mistreatment in your adult relationships as acts of love. Our relationship examples and the level of security we felt around our caregivers molded what we expect and how we behave in relationships as adults.

With all this at play in our psyches, it's no wonder understanding how to navigate a loving commitment with another person can feel overwhelming and confusing. With so much pressure to make your relationship successful or face a lifetime of "incompleteness," it's no wonder we feel terrified of failing. With the narratives of our painful childhood experiences playing out in the background of our minds, it's no surprise we struggle with vulnerability or fear that we are unlovable. It's like going skydiving for the first time and your instructor telling you, "I'm not gonna tell you how to deploy your parachute—you'll have to figure that out midair. Oh, and by the way, you're gonna need to avoid the rocks flying at you." But instead of giving ourselves grace when we find we are caught in unhealthy relationship patterns, we think, *What's wrong with me, why can't I get this right?* Nothing is wrong with you. Relationships are mirrors to the places in us where we are wounded and stuck in the illusion of inadequacy. Unpacking that stuff isn't easy. Your Higher Self knows you deserve all the love, care, support, guidance, and encouragement available to you to keep going. You can do this!

First Things First: Your Partner Does Not Make You Whole

The entire concept of believing your partner completes you is buying into the illusion that you are not complete on our own, that you are not whole. Which is absolutely false. You have always been whole and worthy just for being you. When you buy into that LHB, you will be trapped in the belief that the person who loves you is responsible for your self-worth, and that your partner is no longer an autonomous person on their own journey—they are simply there to make you okay with yourself. And perhaps for a while the relationship does absolve those fears of unworthiness. But inevitably, those old feelings of insecurity and inadequacy, which you hoped your relationship would eradicate, come back. Instead of taking that opportunity to look within, it feels easier to blame the relationship for failing to make you whole. *It must be something my partner isn't giving me,* you think. You switch back and forth between believing you are inadequate to believing your partner is. LHBs are always looking for lack. Your Higher Self knows the truth—**no partner can be another partner's source of self-worth.** And putting that pressure on a relationship only makes the relationship suffer and makes it difficult to embody the love that brought you together in the first place.

We have been made to believe we are lacking in some way and that it's our partner's job to remove that lack through their love. But **love isn't a possession that is given and taken away.** Love is a state of consciousness. It's the awareness of our Higher Selves. The people we love help us open to the awareness of love . . . but they are not the source of love. If we don't connect to our Higher Selves, we easily mistake our partners as the source, believing having a partner is the only path to experiencing the consciousness of love.

Oh boy, was I jealous!

In my early thirties, I dated someone who was different from anyone I'd ever been with. She wasn't an artist; she was a lawyer—which was a big reason I found her attractive. She was a breath of fresh air after dating so many artists. She was responsible, predictable, and seemed…safe.

One evening, we attended a gallery opening, and while I was talking to some friends, I looked over and saw my lawyer girlfriend chatting it up with this girl I vaguely knew. I felt my heart start to race. *What the hell is going on over there? Why are they standing so close together? WTF?*

When we got back to her apartment, I brought it up slowly, asking questions like "Was that Charlotte you were talking to?" "How do you know each other?" "What were you two talking about all that time?" I knew in order to get the truth out of my girlfriend, I couldn't come right out and say, "Just admit you like her!" If there was anything I'd learned from years of watching *Law and Order,* it was that to get a confession, you need to be strategic.

"She's just a friend, Bunny."

She was picking up on what I was trying to insinuate.

But that didn't reassure me. I kept thinking about how Charlotte was a pretty white girl who wore expensive clothing, and probably had a real job with health insurance, while I was this failing artist who shopped at thrift stores and how my girlfriend, the lawyer, would eventually realize I wasn't her type. I needed to keep pushing. I needed to know the truth to protect myself from humiliation.

"Well, maybe you should date Charlotte—I can tell you like her," I snapped.

"Okay, whatever you say," she replied sarcastically.

"Yeah, well, you should! The two of you would be perfect together—you're both assholes!" Then I grabbed my bag and stormed out of her apartment, slamming the door behind me.

Instances like this were common for me in my twenties and early thirties. I'd get paranoid when my partners would give attention to someone I feared was more attractive than me. I'd make snarky remarks or try to pick fights in order to force my partners into proclaiming how much they loved me and/or pleading with me to stay with them.

Those reactions started after I found out my first girlfriend, Kim, had cheated on me. When she went to college in California and I was still a senior at our high school in Texas, we decided to have a long-distance relationship. Over the course of that year, we talked on the phone every day, but little did I know she was secretly sleeping with and in full-on relationships with a series of girls at her college.

At the time I was extremely dependent on Kim emotionally. My parents did not support me when I came out at fifteen, and I believed she was the only person in the world who really loved me for my true self. When I found out about the cheating and the lies, I was devastated. I told myself I would never let that happen again. I'd find someone safe, someone trustworthy.

But no amount of reassurance from my new partners could make me feel safe. No amount of kindness or care prevented my paranoia and jealousy. I'd eventually find myself in a situation where I felt threatened. When I was in that fear state, nothing they did was enough for me.

Behind my jealousy was a deep fear that I was unlovable. I assumed it was because I'd been cheated on, but it began earlier than that. The rejection for being gay from my family, the people who were supposed to love me unconditionally, at such a young age, put the false belief in my head that I wasn't worthy of love.

It took me connecting to my Higher Self to uncover this LHB at the core of my relationships and to give myself grace and compassion for that struggle. Jealousy wasn't a character flaw, and it didn't mean there was something wrong with me. Judging myself for my LHBs was just another form of LHB trying to make me *less than* for struggling.

Understanding that my LHBs are not who I am made it easier to lessen their power over me. Sure, a jealous thought will pop up every now and then, but I now have the practice of asking myself, *What is motivating that thought? Is this an actual situation where my safety in my relationship is being threatened, or is this situation triggering my LHBs because it reminds me of painful experiences from my past?* Perhaps there are knee-jerk reactions that you might have, like my jealousy, that are brought on by LHBs and could perhaps be made less prickly by approaching the situation from the perspective of your Higher Self?

Rethinking Trust

Most of us have had at least one relationship where we felt our trust was violated. Maybe we were cheated on, maybe we were ghosted, maybe a partner hid something from us that they shouldn't have, maybe we grew up in a home where we couldn't depend on the love of our caregivers and we felt neglected or abandoned. No matter the reason, in the aftermath it can feel difficult to know how to repair trust in your relationship or cultivate trust in future relationships.

Someone's inability to be honest in a relationship is not an indication you are unworthy of that honesty; it's an indication that there are underlying issues to be addressed that have nothing to do with your self-worth. Uncovering how those difficult experiences could be motivating you to believe you are somehow inadequate is vital to seeing if a partner is violating the boundaries of your relationship *or* if your LHBs are creating a narrative in your mind that you aren't worthy of love and honesty, therefore leading you to assume you are being treated poorly.

From the Higher Self perspective, cultivating trust for your partner isn't just about the behavior of the person you are in the relationship with. It's also about trusting your own self-worth, and being confident that regardless of the outcome of this relationship, you will always be okay. You are enough. Being grounded in that truth will empower you to let your Higher Self be your guide in making choices out of love, not fear.

Don't Shame Yourself When It Gets Hard

Relationships will inevitably show you your own fears of inadequacy. It takes courage to be accountable and bring those fears out of the unconscious to the conscious — to look at your past wounds, to understand how your LHBs have played a role in undermining your self-worth and the effect that's had on your relationships. Working with a therapist, or partaking in other healing modalities from spiritual practices to self-care, can support the uncovering process.

I want to take this a step further and say, it's not enough to just uncover "your story." You have to realize that you are not your story. Otherwise, you will think to yourself, *I'm not complete until I'm healed of these wounds and triggers.* And your "healing process" becomes another hierarchical belief — another reason to judge yourself and/or your partners as unworthy of love and compassion because of supposed flaws.

Bringing your Higher Self to your relationships isn't just about having compassion for your LHBs; it's also about recognizing that your partner is also dealing with wounds, uncertainty, confusion, Learned Hierarchical Beliefs, and an understanding of relationships based on their past experiences as well. **They come with their "stuff" and you come with yours. But that is not who they are, and it's not who you are either.**

I'm so triggered!

After a particularly difficult fight with Khara, I was in our room, lying in bed and crying while my dog, Rio, whined outside the door. When I was little and heard my parents argue, I wanted to go in their room and yell at them to stop. Now when Khara and I fight, our dog gets anxious and starts biting the furniture or jumping at us to get our attention. My heart rate goes up too, and sometimes I can feel so misunderstood, it feels like my whole world is collapsing.

I pushed my head into the pillow, replaying the fight in my mind. It began after I got upset at Khara for forgetting to lock our back door overnight. When I woke up that morning to meditate and make coffee, I saw that it was unlocked and knew Khara had been the last person to use it.

It made me angry, because Khara knew locking the doors was extremely important to my sense of safety. My indulgence in true crime over the years had lent me an active imagination when it came to being attacked in the middle of the night by an intruder. Plus, growing up, we always locked the door at night—it is just what you are supposed to do!

So the first thing I said when they came down the stairs for coffee wasn't "Good morning, honey, how did you sleep?" It was "You forgot to lock the door *again*."

They got defensive, like I was making too much of a big deal of it. Which only made me feel worse. We went back and forth until I ended the argument by running into our bedroom and slamming the door shut, right after I told them they were "such a jerk."

How could they make light of something so important to me? I thought. *They obviously don't care about my needs and sensitivities—am I that insignificant?*

After twenty minutes of lying in bed, I picked up my phone and opened up TikTok. There was a video of a cat and a dog cuddling together with a super sappy song as the soundtrack. I am a sucker for videos with interspecies love. And that one happened to be cute AF. I noticed my anger and anxiousness subsiding. My heart wasn't pumping out of my chest, and my breathing began to slow down.

I thought about how growing up, I was often told that I was too sensitive, so the moment I think my needs are being diminished, I get triggered and it's really easy for me to be upset.

I also thought about how Khara gets triggered when they feel like they have disappointed me, because growing up they often felt responsible for regulating the emotions of family members.

Then I got a text from them.

> I'm sorry I forgot to lock the door. I promise it won't happen again. I love you so much.

I breathed a sigh of relief and texted them back.

> I'm sorry I called you a jerk. It's ok, I know it's harder for you to remember things like that.

Bringing my Higher Self into the moment helped me see that our argument really wasn't about the door being locked. We were both triggered into old LHBs about not being lovable, and the way to get out of that trap is to connect to our Higher Selves and remember we don't have to stay in that fear place.

Relationships Are Collaborative Healing Projects

Being in a relationship while aligned with your Higher Self is understanding that there is no hierarchy to a person's needs.

Everyone's needs are valid. Our needs are based on where we are in the journey of our own healing. Yes, we are going to be triggered. But **our triggers are not flaws; they are the cues we are working with, the cards we have been dealt.** The more compassionate we are, the less control they have over us. Love is a state of awareness—it's the ability to see the wholeness in ourselves and each other. It's like taking the filter off our LHBs to see our truth. We are all worthy of compassion and understanding. We are all enough just for being who we are. The places that we need to grow are going to rub up against the places that our partners still need to grow. Our relationships are an opportunity to bring conscious awareness to our delusions of inadequacy—which have been ingrained in us by our LHBs and trauma. But they are also a place where we can rewrite our story. That's why relationships are collaborative healing projects!

There Are Many Ways to Be in a Relationship

Every person in a relationship has different needs and boundaries, and that makes a lot of sense because we all come from different experiences and are in different places in our healing journey. For some people monogamy is a relationship structure that feels aligned with their sense of emotional safety, and for others nonmonogamous relationship structures feel more aligned with theirs.

We live in a society that treats monogamy as the moral high ground, and the only answer to finding security in a partnership; but with nearly 50 percent of marriages ending in divorce or separation in the U.S. and infidelity being the second leading cause, it might be high time we question whether monogamy works for everyone.

In her book *Polysecure,* Jessica Fern defines consensual nonmonogamy as "an umbrella term for the practice of simultaneously having multiple partners where everyone involved is aware of and consents to the relationship structure."

There are a lot of misconceptions about consensual non-monogamy, including that people who practice it are simply afraid of commitment or don't really love their partners. And it's quite possible that many people seek out a situation with multiple partners for misguided reasons. It's important to keep in mind that any LHBs you might bring into a monogamous relationship will still show up in a poly one, just manifesting a bit differently. Fern illustrates that although attachment theory is usually written about only in monogamous relationship dynamics, it also applies to polyamorous ones. In other words, being polyamorous does not prevent our wounds from showing up in our committed partnerships, no matter how many partners we have. Having multiple partners doesn't make you more awake to your self-worth—it just changes the format of your journey to discovering it. The same unconscious desire to be completed by one partner can easily become a void that takes multiple partners to fill. Additionally, having one partner does not mean you are able to cultivate more love in your relationship than people who have multiple partners. There are loveless monogamous relationships and loveless non-monogamous ones.

Little by little, alternatives to monogamous paradigms for relationships are entering the mainstream. But ultimately, the structure of your relationship and the level of devotion of your partner or partners will not single-handedly resolve any beliefs of inadequacy or behaviors handed down to you by LHBs.

Whether you are in a monogamous or non-monogamous partnership, loving someone is recognizing their Higher Self and being accountable to your own healing.

A Safe Place for Everyone's Higher Selves

It's incredibly freeing to know that who you really are is separate from the thoughts and behaviors you are working on changing. It's also incredibly freeing for your relationship to remember this is equally true about who you partner with. Connecting to your Higher Self will enable you to love someone for who they really are, their Higher Self—an ever-evolving being who is much more than the role of partner. Someone who has their own needs, desires, dreams, and gifts to share with the world. Just as you are continuing to awaken in your own self-awareness and every day is an opportunity to discover more depth within yourself, it's the same for your partners. As the relationship psychologist Esther Perel so beautifully states in her book *Mating in Captivity,* "The grand illusion of committed love is that we think our partners are ours. In truth, their separateness is unassailable, and their mystery is forever ungraspable."

No matter the obstacles a relationship might face, no matter the LHBs that you are working on unlearning, your Higher Self is always there to bring you back to the awareness of your wholeness and the awareness of your partners. And it's from that consciousness that the partnership will be empowered to grow. Cultivating a safe space for everyone's Higher Selves to shine will light the path for a joyful, peaceful, and bright future.

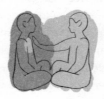

Bring Your Higher Self to Your Committed Relationships

1. **Don't be afraid to look at where your relationship patterns come from.** We all came from a different example of love. Most of us have had difficult past relationships. Bringing our patterns to the surface takes being willing to uncover the beliefs that might be fueling those patterns. Being willing to be

accountable to what you are bringing to the relationship is one of the most loving things you can do, both for yourself and your partners.

2. **Remember, you are not stuck in the past.** As important as it is to unearth childhood wounds so you can heal and understand how they influence your committed partnerships, it's equally (if not more) important to remind yourself that *this* is not your childhood. Your partner is not your mother in another form, or the dad who never showed up. They are not there for you to reenact your past traumas in an attempt to achieve a different outcome. Triggers happen, but managing them is about reminding yourself that you are not that powerless child anymore. You are power-full. You are an adult. You can take care of yourself. You can love freely. You can create your own version of love. The past is not a prison.

3. **You need time alone and autonomy.** A lot of people enter into committed relationships and then stop hanging out with their friends. They give up their hobbies. They stop going dancing. They no longer go on walks alone. It's understandable when you love being around someone so much that you want to be around them all the time. But your Higher Self knows that love comes in many forms. And you deserve to experience it all. On top of that, having space from your partner helps maintain the perspective that without them you would still have support in your life. Your partner cannot be the only well you drink from.

4. **There are many things you don't understand about yourself, so you shouldn't expect your partner to always understand you either.** You both came from different experiences. Not only do we have to be patient with our own journeys toward self-awareness, but we need to be patient and compassionate with our partner's understanding of how best to support us. It's a process. And as long as both of you are committed to showing up for each other, you will grow together in your awareness.

5. **Be willing to evolve and let your partner evolve within the relationship.** Loving someone also means allowing them to grow and evolve as an autonomous person. Loving yourself means allowing yourself to blossom and awaken. In a partnership, this can sometimes take us to places we couldn't have foreseen. But that is natural. A relationship is like a living organism that two people (or more) are nurturing and caring for. The organism needs to evolve to stay alive.

6. **A fight is not a failure.** Conflicts happen. Don't hold yourself up to a standard to handle every conflict with perfect communication. It's just not realistic. The important thing is what you learn from a fight. How did the conflict give you a better understanding of your needs and those of your partners? How can you give yourself more grace? What are some ways you can de-escalate conflicts in the future, both in terms of your personal behavior but also collaboratively with your partner?

7. **Don't stop checking in with each other**. Because we change in our relationships, so do our needs and/or boundaries. Not to mention, life is a roller coaster, and our experiences outside the relationship can also alter our needs. For example, maybe you're anxious about going to your in-laws for the holidays and would like your partner to be a little extra patient and understanding with your moods. Or maybe you are busy with work and your partner would like a better boundary with how much you talk about work at home so the time you spend together is more personal.

   Make it a priority to check in with each other and ask each other, "Is there anything you need from me in terms of support that you're not getting?" or "Can we set aside a time to talk about ways we can create more romance in our relationship?" or "I would like to create a better nighttime schedule with the kids—it hasn't been working well for me." Remember, you are in a collaboration—and when you're building something together, things need to be updated. Just keep in mind, the more centered you are in your Higher Self—the awareness that both of you have valid needs, deserve kindness and compassion, and are still healing from the wounds of the past that shape your emotional experience—the easier it will be to discuss changes and updates that work for both of you.

8. **You are not your partner's therapist and they are not yours.** This one was big for me, because I am obviously very passionate about healing. I get excited to uncover patterns, bring more awareness to Learned Hierarchical Beliefs, and find new ways of reacting to my triggers. So it's easy for me to step into the analytical role with my partner and assume I know why they behave a certain way, then choose the exact *wrong time* to inform them of why they are the way they are—like during an argument. Or I tend to unload my emotions and insecurities about my career or family or friends on my partner and give them an earful during dinner, then expect them to say exactly what I want to hear in response.

    The truth is, there need to be boundaries around our individual healing; and we need support outside of the relationship. When you depend on your partner to guide your healing, you inevitably put too much pressure on the relationship, which can cause the relationship to buckle under the strain.

9. **There is no shame in needing help.** Even though I've always been a proponent of therapy and counseling, I have to admit that when Khara and I first went to couples counseling, there was a part of me that felt ashamed. That part was my LHBs interpreting our need for help as a failure on my part. But seeking help in sustaining a healthy relationship isn't a sign of weakness—it shows strength. It means you value the relationship enough to know you deserve all the help and support you can get. Going to couples counseling was one of the best choices my partner and I could have made for our relationship. I'm so happy I didn't let my shame hold me back.

Relationship Reminders

- Your partner can't read your mind—you have to communicate what you need. Likewise, ask them to communicate their needs. You can't read their mind either.
- A relationship doesn't complete you. It may offer temporary relief from the painful symptoms you experience from not believing you're good enough, but sooner or later, we all have to heal that sh*t ourselves.
- Relationships bring up all the reasons you are afraid you are unlovable. Don't judge yourself if you're having a hard time. This stuff is deep.
- A good partner takes responsibility for projecting their past pain into their present relationship.
- Sometimes what you are angry about in the moment isn't what you are actually hurting from.

Partnership Writing Exercise

Each partner in the relationship writes a description of the other partner's Higher Self (i.e., the different ways you experience your partner's love, light, wisdom, and compassion). This could be a list of loving things they do, how they inspire you, why you appreciate their perspective on the world, what you are learning from them in terms of self-acceptance, and the like. It could be more abstract, like a poem that describes the feelings their Higher Self gives you. There is no right or wrong way. When you are done, share what you wrote with each other.

Journal Prompts

1. Some of my biggest insecurities in my relationship are . . .

2. The past experiences or the beliefs (LHBs) I have grown up with that might be contributing to those fears are . . .

3. Flip the script: My Higher Self would respond to my insecurities by saying . . .

4. The ways my partner(s) shows me kindness and acceptance are . . .

5. The ways I show my partner(s) kindness and acceptance are . . .

6. Some ways I can be more understanding and compassionate in my relationship are . . .

7. Some healthy changes in my relationship I would like to try are . . . (for example: spending less time watching TV, having a monthly check-in on shared finances, setting time every week for a date, having intentional time apart)

8. Things I would like to ask my partner to be more understanding and compassionate of in our relationship are . . .

_____

9. Ways that my partner and I can cultivate more emotional safety when talking about difficult topics are . . .

_____

10. Ways I can show myself more compassion around my relationships are . . .

_____

Chapter 8

Breakups and Being Single

> **Me:** *I feel so rejected by my breakup.*
> **Higher Self:** *That breakup was the Universe telling you you're not compatible. Don't confuse that with rejection.*

———

He dumped me.

Butterflies filled my stomach as I saw my boyfriend, Joey, walking toward my locker in an Alien Workshop T-shirt, baggy pants that revealed plaid boxers underneath, and a silver chain wallet that twinkled in the fluorescent lights of our junior high hallway. Exactly two weeks prior, I had been standing in that exact spot when Joey passed me a note that read:

Will you go out with me? —Joey

Joey was part of what everyone at school called the biker posse: a group of popular eighth- and ninth-grade boys who rode around the neighborhood on BMX bikes, wearing JNCO jeans and smoking stogies (what everyone cool called cigarettes).

I wrote back, "Yes."

The two weeks of our relationship thus far had consisted mostly of awkward phone conversations and two times fooling around in his den while listening to Bone Thugs's *East 1999 Eternal.*

Joey now approached my locker and without making eye contact, passed me a note and kept walking. My stomach dropped. I quickly turned toward my locker, shielding myself with the door, like a turtle trying to get back into its shell. In my makeshift cave, I unfolded the note slowly, deciphering Joey's barely legible chicken scratch:

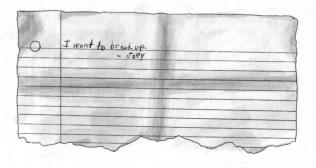

"Oh my God, Joey dumped you?" my friend Edie asked when she approached me as I waited to order chicken fingers in the lunch line. I'd managed not to cry during the two classes I'd had since I got his breakup note. I felt humiliated, but I didn't want anyone to see me upset in case word got back to Joey.

"Where did you hear that?" I asked.

"Like, from a lot of people. Joey told everyone he dumped you in a note. God, I'm really sorry."

To avoid Edie's half-sympathetic, half-mirthful facial expression,

I turned my gaze toward the trash cans by the door, full of plastic forks, leftover tater tots, used ketchup packets, and empty Capri Suns. The sign above it read, STUDENTS: DUMP ALL TRASH IN THE PROPER RECEPTACLES. This was my first time getting dumped, but I knew what it meant. I was the trash. I was the loser. And now everyone knew it.

Breakups Are Not Failures

I'm sure most of you reading this book have gone through a breakup where at the time it felt like the worst possible thing you could be experiencing, and then years later you looked back at that time in your life and thought, *Thank God I got out of that relationship!*

But that doesn't change the fact that when it happens, it hurts. The short-lived love affairs in junior high sting, but the breakups of relationships you'd hoped would last forever — the ones where you felt truly in love — those are excruciating. Not only are you grieving the companionship of that person, but you are grieving the loss of the expectations you had for that relationship. You're grieving the routine you had as a couple, the plans you made, the friends you shared, the things you enjoyed doing together — these separations throw all aspects of our identities into question. *Do I even like anchovies on my pizza?* Suddenly it feels like you don't know who you are.

And then there are the physiological effects. According to the American anthropologist Helen Fischer, who researched the effects of romantic love on the brain, the same part of your brain that becomes activated with motivation, craving, and drive when you fall in love craves even more when that attachment is taken away. In other words, when you feel heartbroken, your brain is in overdrive to get that relationship back. A brain scan of a person who recently experienced the loss of romantic love will look very similar to a person who is going through cocaine or opioid withdrawal. Which is part of why you feel tempted to text your ex or look them up on social media—your brain is trying to get its fix.

Wouldn't it be great if when we decided we want to get over a relationship, it would just magically happen? Perhaps that's why the plot of the film *Eternal Sunshine of the Spotless Mind,* in which people could hire a service to wipe away all memories of a past lover, resonated with so many people.

But what makes a breakup, separation, or divorce even more difficult is that our culture has set us up to believe that when it happens, it means something went terribly wrong. That the relationship failed. That you or your ex must suffer from some inadequacy.

Throughout Western culture, the "failure" of a marriage has been equated with moral failure and the freedom to divorce was controlled by patriarchal and religious hierarchies. The Roman Catholic Church defined marriage as a holy sacrament and prohibited the legalization of divorce in Catholic countries for centuries. The Protestant Reformation saw marriage as more of a social contract than a theological one; however, Protestant women had no legal rights to divorce. Shockingly, it wasn't until 2010 that every state in the United States passed no-fault divorce laws granting a divorce based on irreconcilable differences.

And then there are the pressures many of us felt from our families and/or parental figures to find a husband or a wife and have children—so the consequences of a breakup are compounded by the disappointment of your loved ones who are anxiously waiting for you to "settle down."

Our culture sees romantic relationships from a hierarchical lens (you're not enough if you don't have one)—and it sees breakups that way as well. When you are taught that you need to find one person to be with "until death do you part," why wouldn't you see the ending of a relationship as an omen for a life of loneliness and misery? Why wouldn't you believe that until you find someone new, you won't be complete?

Our Learned Hierarchical Beliefs that breakups equal failure—whether your failure, your partner's, or the relationship's—make it more difficult to allow ourselves to grieve and repair our broken hearts, to learn from past relationships, and to know when a breakup is exactly what's needed. Lots of people will stay in unhappy relationships just to avoid the pain, shame, or embarrassment of a relationship ending. And often the consequences are devastating; in some cases, even dangerous.

My breakup was my breakthrough.

One day when I was twenty-five years old, I ran out of my basement apartment in south Brooklyn and the sunshine shocked me like the flash of a Polaroid camera. After my momentary blindness, the beautiful spring day came into focus and I observed my bustling neighborhood: teenagers hanging out on a stoop, a mom pushing a baby carriage, a girl with spiky green hair hurrying to catch the M train. It was an entirely different reality from what I was walking out of.

My partner and I had been fighting for hours, culminating in him hitting me and me running out our front door. Now I was standing outside, frozen, face puffy from crying, blood on the side of my cheek, and I had no idea what to do. I had no money. I didn't even have a cell phone because I shared one with my partner and I had left it with him. I was worried he might hurt himself.

Just walk. Just get out of here.

I crossed Broadway and went into the bodega with the neon Halal sign.

"Can I please borrow some change to make a phone call?" I asked the guy behind the counter who normally sold me

Parliament Lights and the occasional breakfast sandwich. I was trying to hold back tears.

Without saying a word, he graciously slid over two quarters. I walked to the side of the building and called my friend on the payphone. She said she would be right there. I hung up and waited. I felt a sting from salty tears dripping into the wound on the side of my cheek.

I was used to concentrating emotional pain to one area of my body rather than having it floating inside me aimlessly, like a balloon released into the sky.

My friend's truck pulled up on the curb. Thank God she got there fast. If it had taken much longer, I probably would have gone back home.

Once we were out of my neighborhood, I could finally take a deep breath. *This is the end of my relationship,* I decided. At a red light, I looked out the window and saw a cherry tree. It had just begun to bud.

I never would have guessed that I was about to enter a time in my life that in some ways was more challenging than the five years I had spent in an abusive relationship.

The breakup felt like jumping into a freezing cold lake, chilling me to the bone and turning me inside out. I couldn't hide from myself anymore. I had to confront loneliness, isolation, fear, depression, anger, and humiliation. I had to look in the mirror and ask myself, "How did I get here?" I had to resist running back into my partner's arms, the place I had called home for so long. The worst part about it was that once I fully comprehended the abuse, I felt I could no longer trust myself to make choices that were good for me.

I realize now that my Higher Self had been there the whole time, speaking to me through my heart, setting off alarm bells that I was unsafe. Only I wasn't ready to listen. I silenced that voice. I didn't tell my friends and family what was going on, because I knew it was wrong. I drank and did drugs to avoid my true feelings.

It wasn't that I couldn't trust myself—the lesson was the opposite. I needed to trust myself more. I needed to listen to my Higher Self—the wisdom within me that had always known what I really deserve.

You're Still Learning from Your Ex

Breakups do not actually end the relationship. They just change the form of it.

You are still in a relationship with all of your exes, because they have taught you about what you want and what you don't want in a partner. They held up a mirror to your fears, wounds, hopes, and vulnerabilities. That's what relationships do. If you are willing to let them, they help you grow, by using those experiences to your advantage—for example, becoming aware of behavior patterns that no longer serve you, red flags you didn't pay attention to, and boundaries you realize you need in a partnership. You carry those lessons with you into all your future relationships. Only now, you won't be learning from each other together, you will be learning from each other apart. Everything that happens is part of the curriculum of awakening to your Higher Self—the part of you that knows your worth. If you are going through a breakup, it is the breakthrough that you need.

Why Rejection Isn't Real

From the Higher Self perspective, there is no such thing as rejection. Rejection implies a loss of acceptance or approval. But your Higher Self knows that acceptance and approval come from within, not without. There is no such thing as someone who is capable of rejecting you—because you are enough just for being you.

If someone doesn't want to be in a relationship with you it's not because you are not enough for them, it's because your paths are no longer aligning. And that could be for a number of reasons. And no, it doesn't feel good to learn that someone you want to be with, someone you love, needs to go their separate way. But if their path is leading them a different way, that means they can no longer give you what you need. Similarly, staying with someone because you don't want to hurt them is not a loving thing to do. You can't give them what they need, so why are you holding on? Are you protecting them or are you running away from honesty and accountability? Caring for someone does not always mean staying together. Love guides us often to make difficult choices. Breakups can be an act of love.

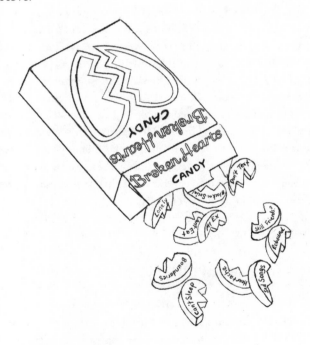

Grieving a Relationship

Our culture puts a lot of pressure on us to "get over" our romantic relationships quickly, to prove to ourselves and to others that we are okay. And it's more convenient than ever to just log on to a dating app and try to distract yourself from your feelings. (Hello, rebounds.)

In a patriarchal society, feeling your feelings, admitting you are in pain, and being vulnerable are seen as signs of weakness. If you were really strong, if you were really good enough, you would be over it, right? You wouldn't be at home crying, ordering takeout for the fifth day in a row, getting nauseous every time you think of your ex with another person.

But letting yourself grieve is a necessary process of understanding what the ending of this relationship is teaching you about your own self-acceptance. Whenever I hear "I want to get over it," I imagine a person jumping over a big pile of dirty laundry on their floor, thinking that will get their clothes clean.

Letting yourself grieve is feeling your feelings without rushing to change them, denying they exist, or believing there is something wrong with you for having them. You have to hang out with that big pile of dirty laundry on your floor. It's ugly, it's smelly, it's taken over your entire bedroom. Some days you go out with your friends and have a good time only to come back home and find it's still there, waiting for you. This will last until eventually you begin sorting through each piece, deciding which clothes are worth putting in the wash and which need to be thrown out. You can think of this process as building awareness about what beliefs you want to hold on to about that relationship, and which ones you want to let go of.

For example, do I want to take away from this relationship the belief that all men are horrible, or that because it didn't work out, I won't find love again? Or do I want to take away from this relationship the belief that I grew from the experience, that I learned what didn't work for me?

It's a tedious process, but because you are patient and compassionate, you get through it. And you get your room back. **We can't foretell how something ending in our lives marks a new and necessary beginning.** That perspective doesn't come until enough time has passed for reflection. Showing up for your own grief is a sacred process of alchemizing your pain into a deeper sense of self-acceptance and wisdom.

You are guaranteed to bring the experiences of your past relationships into your new ones. The question is, do you want to do that consciously or unconsciously? Do you do it in ways that hinder your happiness or in ways that support it?

Villainizing Your Ex Is a Form of Dependence

Anger is a useful emotion. It can wake us up to realizing things need to change. It can soothe us when we feel hurt. Getting together with your friends after a hard breakup and talking shit about your ex can make you feel better. *"God, what an asshole! You are so much better without him!"* your friends tell you over a round of margaritas, and it feels great to have that support.

We have all secretly checked our ex's social media hoping they are not doing well without us. But needing your ex to be suffering without you is just another form of needing validation from them. Only this time it's not coming from their love; it's coming from their misery. This behavior can escalate to extreme levels. Think about the millions of dollars spent in divorce proceedings fighting over possessions that ultimately do not matter or make you any happier. It happens because some people would rather spend an enormous amount of money, resources, and their own time rather than let their exes "win."

Sadly, a lot of breakups become competitions of who is the better, more deserving person. Which is unsurprising in a hierarchical belief system in which we are constantly measuring ourselves against each other. If our relationship gives us status and self-worth, its breakup takes that away. We feel diminished by our ex-partners, so what do we do? We try to diminish them to feel better about ourselves.

Ultimately, this reinforces the belief that your worth is dependent on how your ex feels. Constant comparisons only make it harder to focus on yourself, your healing, and the realization that in or out of the relationship, you have always been enough.

No matter what mistakes they have made, your ex is a person just like you, one with their own set of Learned Hierarchical Beliefs, their own wounds, and their own struggle for self-acceptance. Hating them or wanting to take revenge isn't a sustainable way to feel better. Hoping that they get the healing they need while knowing that is not your responsibility will free you from unhealthy attachment.

When YOU Want to Break Up

When I broke up with Noah, the boy I had lost my virginity to and who had been my boyfriend for almost three years by the time I was fourteen, he cried so much that when my dad saw us sitting in the back patio, Noah wiping the tears from his face with the collar of his Grateful Dead T-shirt, my dad couldn't help but cry too. Two days later, Noah intentionally overdosed on Tylenol and was taken to the emergency room. When I came to visit him, I sat by his bed while he had to eat crushed-up charcoal in a Styrofoam cup. The black particles covered his teeth and sent a chill down my spine as he looked up to me and asked, "Now can we get back together?"

For many years I held on to that guilt. If I hadn't broken up with him, he wouldn't have tried to take his own life, or ended up in a mental health hospital afterward. At the time, Noah's parents were going through a divorce and he was struggling with drug addiction and an undiagnosed mental health crisis; the breakup had just been the icing on the cake. It didn't matter, though—that experience made me terrified of hurting anyone again.

So how do we break up with people when we know it will hurt them?

The first thing we need to keep in mind is that if we have decided to end a relationship, that means we have had a lot more time to process that it's ending than our partner has. We have been going through the reality of a breakup in our own head for some time and have come to the conclusion this is what is best for us. But our partner has not had that advantage. They don't know what is coming. So we can and should expect some pushback, difficult emotions, and reactivity. It's only human. We cannot expect it not to hurt.

The second thing we need to be aware of is that breaking up isn't just about you not getting what you need from the relationship any longer; it's about you not being able to give that person what they need either. If it's not right for you, it's not right for them. Relationships are unsustainable without mutual commitment.

And the third thing is that just because there are hurt feelings doesn't mean that anyone is doing anything wrong. In actuality, you are doing something right; breakups are an act of love. It does not serve the person you care about to stay with them when you are unhappy.

Ultimately there is no getting around the heavy feelings and loss of expectations that the dissolution of a relationship can induce. But your Higher Self knows that you are on a path of self-realization. That path isn't always a smooth ride, but it's not supposed to be. When we lose something we hold dear, what we are left with is ourselves. It's a chance to see what a gift we truly are. As the psychologist Katherine Woodward Thomas writes in her book *Conscious Uncoupling: Five Steps to Living Happily Ever After*, "In a nutshell, a breakup is nothing short of a once-in-a-lifetime opportunity to have a complete spiritual awakening. One that catapults you to a whole new level of authenticity, compassion, wisdom, depth, and—dare I say it?—even joy."

Single Life

I remember playing this card game when I was little called Old Maid. The object of the game was to make as many pairs as you could, and whoever was left with the odd queen card was the Old Maid and lost the game. I asked my older sister what an old maid was and she said, "It's a woman who never gets married and has to live alone her whole life." "The worst possible fate for a woman" is what I took away from that. There should have been another card game where the loser ended up trapped in an unhappy marriage for the rest of their life, if you ask me.

In every Disney movie, rom-com, and teenybopper sitcom, having a "person" was a marker for success and a happy ending. Even the movies that are somewhat progressive about the cultural bias against singledom—the judgment from friends and family, the fears of getting older and not finding someone—fall short of revising this definition. Take *Bridget Jones's Diary*, for example. Her transformation happens when despite the judgment and stigma she feels for being single, she starts accepting herself for who she is—and her reward for this is that she finds "the one." How radical would it have been if the happy ending had been Bridget alone in her apartment, the British voiceover saying, "And in the end I realized I don't need a bloody man to be happy."

In America, married people have privileges that single people do not. There are more than one thousand laws that financially benefit married couples over single people, including tax breaks and health care benefits. Politicians routinely refer to their constituents as working families, even though according to the census bureau in 2021, nearly half of the U.S. population is single. One can only presume that these politicians are speaking to the assumption that the goal of single people is to eventually have a family.

Being single comes with the stigma of rejection or possessing some sort of energetic block that keeps you from finding "the one." Your life is in a state of limbo or hasn't really begun. "When are you going to settle down?" your aunt asks you at Thanksgiving while passing you the mashed potatoes. "I have this coworker I want to set you up with!" your friend from yoga class texts you. When you tell someone you are going through a divorce, they reply, "Oh God, I am so, so sorry," as if it is the absolute worst possible thing that could be happening. In a world of haves and have-nots, romance is a status symbol and singledom is a state of lack. So it makes sense that being single can feel like something is missing or something is wrong. Because in a very real way, what is missing is the respect our society should have for single people. What is missing is you letting yourself be enough.

Many people all over this world are not looking for a romantic partner, either because it's not what they want for this time in their life, or because they just flat out feel happier living single.

And let's not forget about people who identify as aromantic. Aromanticism is an identity that covers a spectrum of experiences including folks who feel little to no romantic connection to others, and people who feel more aligned with other forms of intimacy that they would not describe as romantic.

Even if you are not single by choice and are searching for your next romantic relationship, dismantling the stigma you have internalized about something being wrong with you is essential to finding peace during this time—however short or long term it is.

Your Higher Self empowers you to notice when LHBs put narratives in your mind that you are inadequate for being single. When those thoughts come up, remind yourself that relationship status—whether single, married, or dating—does not have to determine the state of your happiness.

Feeling Lonely

I don't know about you, but when I start feeling lonely, I often catch myself internalizing it as a personal failing. Like, *If I was cooler I'd have more friends*, or, *If I was lovable, I would always feel loved*, or, *If people really liked me, then they would be texting me all the time*. But loneliness isn't always about being alone. That is why people who are surrounded by others all the time can still feel lonely. Loneliness can often be about not feeling seen by other people as our authentic selves. This leads us to believe that we are actually alone in our experience. Then we get into a cycle of convincing ourselves that we are truly alone: We stop reaching out to other people, energetically close our hearts, and isolate ourselves. This feeds into more feelings of loneliness, and the cycle continues.

We also live in a very individualistic culture that doesn't prioritize mutual care, a society that often leaves people to fend for themselves, where a sense of community and even humanity can seem out of reach. But all of us want the same thing—to feel loved and accepted. We are the opposite of being alone in that experience. The sooner you realize this, the sooner you will realize that offering your friendship and companionship is a sacred gift—and how deserving you are of receiving love yourself.

Every person needs connection. It's what makes us human. And we all feel lonely from time to time. But being lonely is not the same as solitude. We get lonely when we start to believe we don't deserve connection. When you are in solitude, you might be physically separated from other people, but you are aware of the fact that you can never truly be alone. Your heart is part of our interconnected consciousness: You are one with other people, as well as the trees, the stars, the animals, the ocean, the wind...Some of my most profound moments of connectedness to others I have experienced in solitude—sitting in meditation, feeling at one with all creation.

It's easy to feel lonely after a breakup, because the person who used to be there—beside you on the couch or texting you on the phone or lying with you in bed—is gone. The solitude you have been thrust into can feel like an indication that you are not okay. What is really happening is that you have entered a state of transition and you need to make adjustments to your new circumstances.

I have a theory as to why it is so hard for some of us to be alone post-breakup. It's that we get social anxiety with ourselves. If we haven't spent any quality time with ourselves in a long time because we were always with our partner, we don't know how to have a good time alone—same as with any stranger. If we can avoid being alone, the result is that we avoid getting to know ourselves.

Think about it: You go from spending all this time with one person—cooking dinner, watching movies, making plans, relaxing on days off, and so on, to now spending much more time alone. You don't know what makes you happy. You don't know your motivations, what inspires you, what your wounds are, and what you need to work on healing.

It's incredibly difficult to build self-awareness if you don't prioritize being with yourself. And these days it's easier than ever to avoid being with yourself, even if you are physically alone. You can just go on your phone, watch Netflix, play a video game — all of which are totally fine. There is nothing wrong with doing any of these activities. But there is another kind of alone time — "quality" alone time — that is absolutely necessary.

Think about it as any other relationship: You know there is a difference between watching TV on the couch with your partner and going on a hike together or having a meaningful conversation. Yes, when you are watching TV you are spending time together, but you aren't really connecting. It's the same with our relationship to ourselves.

Relationships need nurturing to thrive. But you won't know how to nurture yourself if you avoid learning your own needs. In a system of Learned Hierarchical Beliefs that has us constantly reaching for outside validation, our most important relationship often gets put on the back burner: our relationship with ourselves, where we can cultivate and connect to our Higher Selves. And guess what? When we avoid knowing ourselves, that means that even if we find another relationship, we won't know what our needs in that relationship really are, and we are likely to fall back into the trap of self-avoidance.

Prioritizing being a good partner to yourself helps you distinguish between when you need to spend time with other people and when some time in solitude will be good for you.

Your Higher Self is accessible through an inner dimensional shift. In order to be on the path toward aligning with your Higher Self, you need to prioritize honoring your time alone. Whether you are in a relationship or not.

Staying Friends

A common question from listeners of my podcast, *XO Higher Self*, is whether they should remain friends with their ex. I always ask the same question back: Are you really *just* friends? If your ex started a new romance with someone else, would you be able to hear about it or even hang out with their new person the way you would with another friend?

A relationship that has gone from romantic to platonic does not automatically transfer to the status of "just friends." Even if friendship is ultimately the goal, you should always take some time apart first. The reason it is good to take some distance from your ex after a breakup is that it's very hard to see the Higher Self perspective on the breakup while you are still looking at it from the inside out.

Often when we stay close with our exes, we unconsciously bring the same grievances, anger, and wounds with us to the new platonic relationship, hoping that someday the dynamic between you two will change enough for all that unpleasant stuff to go away. We look for healing in the same relationship we need to heal from.

Creating a boundary from your ex and taking space makes it easier to see what happened from the Higher Self perspective—which is like a bird's-eye view, or understanding from a higher state of consciousness.

Without that perspective, knowing whether a friendship with this person is in your own best interest will be almost impossible. Remember, making decisions based on what you think your Higher Self would want you to do isn't always easy. Often it is the more challenging choice. Because unlearning, healing, and awakening to your self-worth isn't easy. If it was, everyone would be doing it, because the payoff is a more joyful authentic life.

Happy and Wanting a Relationship

It is possible to be happy being single while wanting a relationship at the same time. Yup, just like it's possible to be happy in your graduate program or at an internship while knowing you want to land a great job afterward. The path of your Higher Self is knowing you are enough right now. This doesn't mean you don't have wants or desires; it just means that your self-acceptance isn't put on the back burner until you get what you want. All through life, we will have times when we get what we want and times when we don't. Life is full of ups and downs. Aligning with your Higher Self is knowing that your worth isn't dependent on what happens. Why put your self-acceptance in the hands of circumstances that are so often beyond your control?

Contrary to what we have been told our whole lives, your relationship status, whether single, newly broken up, or partnered up, ultimately is not the determining factor of your self-worth. And the sooner you realize that, the sooner you will make choices that reflect what really feels right to you and what you really deserve. The sooner you will be able to enjoy each day, knowing you have permission to experience joy no matter what.

No matter how challenging a breakup is, you will get through it. And your Higher Self will always be there to guide you forward.

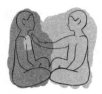

Find Your Higher Self in Romantic Breakups

1. **Investigate the LHBs being triggered by the breakup that are about more than the relationship.** A breakup is a triggering experience. And a lot of the pain comes from fears and insecurities that go deeper than what is happening now. For example, feelings of unworthiness from experiencing abandonment in childhood or a cultural belief that you should be married by this time. Bringing that stuff to your awareness will help you be more empowered in managing those difficult feelings. You can remind yourself, *I'm triggered right now. That is why this is extra painful. But triggers don't last forever. I will be okay.*

2. **Ask for support.** No one should have to go through a breakup without love from friends and family. But a lot of people do. So many of us are ashamed to call up a friend and say, "Hey, I'm having a hard time, I need some support." This is especially true if we haven't sought the support of people outside our relationship for a long time. A big LHB in our culture is that vulnerability is weakness. So yeah, it's gonna feel scary to get out of your comfort zone and ask for help when you need it. Likewise, if someone you care about is going through a breakup, make sure to let them know you are there for them, and keep checking in. It might be difficult for them to reach out.

3. **Healing is a balance of compassion and encouragement.** Aligning with your Higher Self means embodying self-compassion and self-acceptance with a willingness to keep

growing, unlearning, and healing. It's a balance between kindness and encouragement. Between stillness and action. Your process of grieving the ending of your relationship is going to take time. But actively giving yourself the tools and putting yourself in supportive environments is how you keep moving forward. For example, looking at your ex's Instagram is understandable when you miss them or you want to know what they have been up to, but on a deeper level your heart knows that it doesn't help your healing journey and doesn't make you feel good. So it's not about shaming yourself for wanting to look (your Higher Self does not shame); it's about acknowledging, "Okay, I want to do this, and it's understandable that I do, but looking at their Instagram will not actually help me. So let me see if I can get through the day without looking." Again, it's a balance of being present in self-compassion while still encouraging yourself to dig deep.

4. **Create a list of breakup boundaries.** In Alcoholics Anonymous, people who are in the process of getting sober are encouraged to not set foot in a bar, even if they plan on drinking soda. Why? Because when tempted in the moment, it's hard to make the right decision. The end of a relationship is the same. Why make it harder by engaging in activities that don't help you? You need boundaries. Everyone's boundaries are going to look different. If you are ever unsure about a boundary, ask yourself if engaging in that behavior is helping your healing or hindering it. Likewise, always respect your ex's boundaries—even if they feel like a punch in the gut. Once, after a really difficult breakup, one of my exes cut off contact with me and I totally freaked out. I called her multiple times in a row, texted over and over again, left voicemails crying and begging her to talk to me. She didn't budge. Now I realize that was the best thing that could have happened in that moment. I will be forever grateful that she had the strength to set that boundary, because it was so necessary for me to move past my attachment to her.

Here are some examples of breakup boundaries: blocking your ex's Instagram so you can't see their pictures; not texting or talking on the phone with your ex; if there is something that needs to be discussed, doing it through email so you aren't tempted to get reactive. Not going to a party your ex is attending. Not listening to any sad breakup songs or watching romantic movies that make you upset. If you are going through a difficult divorce and have to discuss logistics or schedules for children, do it with a mediator, such as a therapist or family counselor.

Make sure to write out a list of your boundaries rather than just having them in your head. It will help you commit. And if you fall off or break a boundary, don't beat yourself up about it; you can start fresh tomorrow. These boundaries might change over time as you tend to your healing and need different things.

Affirmation Spell for Lessening Attachment to an Ex

If you are really struggling in your breakup, I'd recommend doing this spell every day for at least two weeks. Otherwise, do it whenever you are having a difficult time or stuck in sad thoughts about the breakup, such as hearing news about them with a new partner, or whenever you feel called to.

- Get a light-colored candle, preferably white, that has never been lit before. This candle is going to be used for the purpose of this spell only.
- Find a quiet spot where you will not be interrupted.
- Light the candle.
- Close your eyes and repeat this affirmation ten times:
- "I wish you, _____(your ex's name), health and healing, but your journey is no longer my responsibility."
- Open your eyes and blow out the candle.

Journal Prompts

1. The LHBs that are influencing my perspective on my breakup are...

   _____

2. Flip the script: My Higher Self would tell me this about my breakup...

   _____

3. I can give myself more compassion around my difficult feelings by...

   _____

4. Changes in my behaviors and/or boundaries that will help me better process my breakup are...

   _____

5. What I have learned from my breakups thus far is...

   _____

6. Being single is not failing at relationships because...

   _____

7. Some things I can do to take myself out on a date are...

   _____

Chapter 9

Friendship

> **Me:** *I have no friends. No one ever calls or texts me.*
> **Higher Self:** *Have you called or texted anyone? In order to have friends, you have to be a friend.*

My bosom friend

In the book *Anne of Green Gables,* the main character, Anne Shirley, describes her best friend, Diana Berry, as "a bosom friend—a real kindred spirit to whom I can confide my innermost soul." My best friend in elementary school, Catherine, reminded me of Diana Berry. Or at least the actress who played Diana Berry in the made-for-TV film version. She had the same long dark hair, pale skin, and rosy cheeks. From the fifth to seventh grade, we were inseparable. My parents liked Catherine too. My mom even let me go on vacations to her family's beach house in Galveston.

Catherine lived in a big house, but she never made me feel weird about it. We had so many firsts together—first boyfriends, first cigarette, first period, first time going to the mall and the movies without a parent coming with us. Once we drank a whole bunch of Jolt soda because we heard it had the most caffeine of any soda and pretended that we were drunk. Our favorite thing was to bake a box of brownies and eat nearly the entire tray.

On birthdays, we had a tradition of making each other a big collage that was an ode to our friendship. There would be cut-outs from magazines of our favorite movies like *Romeo and Juliet* (the Claire Danes and Leonardo DiCaprio version), pictures of our favorite musicians like TLC or Alanis Morrisette, and mementos from things we did together, like the ribbon from the matching princess crowns we got at Scarborough Fair.

Then, the summer after seventh grade, I kissed Catherine's ex-boyfriend, Chase. They had just broken up a few weeks prior, and Catherine was upset about the breakup — in fact, she was hoping they would get back together. The three of us were at Catherine's family's beach house, celebrating her birthday. We spent the day swimming at the beach, and I noticed Chase flirting with me right in front of Catherine. It took me by surprise. I thought if he liked me, then I was pretty and interesting, possibly more pretty and interesting than Catherine. I believed that attention from boys was confirmation you were good enough. Later that night, the three of us were hanging out on the deck looking at the stars. Catherine went inside to get us something to drink, and Chase put his arm around me, so I leaned over and kissed him. Right at that moment, Catherine walked out and caught us. All she did was go to her room. The following day was Catherine's actual birthday. The plan was to go to Golden Corral for breakfast. But instead, her mom pulled me and Chase aside and said she was sending us to the airport, that I had really hurt Catherine's feelings.

I tried to apologize, but Catherine never talked to me again. The next year, she went to a private school, so we stopped running into each other. I have not seen or talked to Catherine since her birthday at the beach house.

I wish I had known how special that friendship was at the time, and how much more important it was than being "chosen" by a boy. I also think my LHBs related to my family having less money and not being a white girl and therefore "less" attractive than Catherine were also part of my motivation to compete with her.

In *Anne of Green Gables,* Diana's mom refuses to let her be friends with Anne anymore after a misunderstanding makes her think Anne got Diana drunk. And when Diana secretly meets up with Anne to give her the news that they can no longer be friends, they both cry and Anne takes a lock of Diana's dark hair for a keepsake, pledging that even though they can no longer be together, she will always remain her bosom friend. I still hold a special place in my heart for my bosom friend, Catherine.

Barriers to Making Friends

Everyone agrees that friendship is an important part of a healthy childhood. Children are encouraged to be social; in fact, the more friends you have (i.e., the more popular you are), the better. But for a lot of us, making friends, even when we were young, wasn't easy.

This is especially true if you were ostracized or bullied due to your physical appearance, race, sex, disability, or class; maybe you are neurodivergent and communicated differently than most of your classmates, making the social experience of school even more challenging. Most of us carry those beliefs into our adulthood— about whether we deserve supportive friends and community or feel open to meeting and getting to know new people.

And then there are our culture's hierarchical beliefs about what kind of relationships are most important. Non-romantic relationships aren't given as much social and cultural priority as romantic ones. The purpose of non-romantic friendship is support, love, and companionship; those virtues are not important in a hierarchical society that teaches you that you need to compete with others to be successful. So why wouldn't you see your friends as competition rather than community? Why wouldn't it be intuitive to deprioritize friendships once you are in a romantic relationship?

In a society where your worth is equal to your productivity, it also makes sense that work and career would take precedence over social life. When it's ingrained in you that marriage and kids are the keys to your happiness, staying home and cooking dinner for your family instead of catching up with a friend you haven't seen in months makes sense. It would be nice, but it's not that important, right?

In Lydia Denworth's book *Friendship: The Evolution, Biology, and Extraordinary Power of Life's Fundamental Bond,* she illustrates one reason why little scientific research has been done on friendship and social bonds compared to romantic and familial relationships: It is because biologists did not see friendships as having any influence on reproduction. I would also argue that because friendships

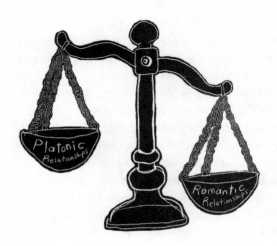

were not seen as integral to upholding Western ideals of prosperity through the accumulation of wealth and status, it's not surprising that Western medicine didn't put it high on its to-do list either.

LHBs about our own inadequacy when it comes to our physical appearance, race, class, or career success make us feel socially insecure—afraid to try to form friendships with people we perceive as "better" than us in some way. *They wouldn't want to be friends with me,* we often tell ourselves. We see friend groups out at bars or on social media and believe that if we were as cool, attractive, and successful as those people, we would also be surrounded by a bunch of close friends. *I must not be good enough to have that.*

Competition Rather Than Community

Have you ever noticed that the people you envy most, when you see them post their successes on social media, or doggedly pursuing their career goals and passions, are very often people you have the most in common with? People with the same interests, dreams, and desires? When our culture teaches us to measure our worth through comparing ourselves to other people, it makes sense that we would feel threatened when someone we relate to seems to be doing "better" than us. Because of this, instead of seeing this similar person as a potential friend, they become an enemy. According to our Learned Hierarchical Beliefs, you can't be good enough unless you are better than someone else.

When we see the world through this competitive lens, it's easy to feel alone and isolated. It's easy to shy away from building mutually supportive relationships, from taking part in community or believing that anyone wants you to succeed or cares about you. Our LHBs keep us from seeing the goodness in other people, from having compassion or even genuine interest in their experience other than how it makes us look. They also keep us from seeing our own inherent value where we assume other people would have little interest in getting to know us. When others become mirrors to project the delusion that we are inadequate, it's easier to isolate.

It's true that having social connections and making friends isn't easy for everyone — especially when you socially relate differently, or if you didn't pick up those skills growing up. But often, our greatest psychic blocks to connection are our unconscious LHBs.

But in the pursuit of success, independence, and self-sufficiency, we have nearly lost one of the most important truths of our human existence: We need each other, and we also need to feel a sense of belonging.

Too old to make friends?

One busy Monday morning, I took a break from working on this book and opened up Instagram stories. Right away, I saw a bunch of photos from an acquaintance's birthday party over the weekend. I felt a pain in my stomach. *I wish I had been invited.* The more I scrolled, the more I saw from other friends who had been invited, laughing, dancing, looking like they were having the greatest time at the coolest party. A familiar LHB started to sink in. *If I was cooler or more interesting, I'd have more friends.*

Six months before, I had moved to upstate New York from NYC and was feeling increasingly isolated. I'd had the same two best friends for years, and now they were hundreds of miles away. Even though I would consider my spouse, Khara, to also be my best friend, I know it's not the same as a close platonic bond.

I was nearly forty, and the idea of making a new friend seemed increasingly difficult. I'd think about how when we were little kids, it was totally natural for some other little kid to come up to you in the sandbox and ask, "Will you be my friend?" I'd imagine myself going up to someone at the Village Coffee shop in my town and asking that. They'd probably think,

Can I just drink my oat milk latte in peace without this weirdo bothering me?

There was someone I'd met a couple of times briefly in the city, and who I had seen on Instagram also moved upstate recently. *Should I send her a DM and see if she wants to hang out sometime?* I thought to myself. I looked up her profile and did a quick scan of the pictures she'd posted, trying to get a sense if she was too busy or if she might reject me. *Oh my god, I'm so nervous, it's like I'm in my twenties again, asking someone on a date!*

When we let our Learned Hierarchical Beliefs unconsciously run our lives, we are used to seeing other people through a lens of "Are they better than me or am I better than them?" Being open to connecting with other people requires connecting to your Higher Self, who knows no one is better than you and that you are no better than anyone else. Most of the time we walk around assuming people are judging us, which really means we are judging *them*. Making a friend or becoming closer to a friend you already have requires vulnerability. Letting yourself be vulnerable with someone is an act of love for yourself, because you are affirming that your feelings and experience are important and worthy of sharing.

Our friendship is one of the greatest gifts we have to offer someone. When we start seeing our own value, then we begin to recognize the value we bring to other people's lives.

After about ten minutes of trying to decide exactly how to word my DM to this potential new friend, I finally sent it.

> Hi! How are you? Not sure if you remember, but we met a few months ago at our mutual friend's birthday party. I saw that you recently moved upstate from the city. So did I! I would love to meet up for coffee or a drink sometime. Looking for some local friends;)

Sent.

I quickly closed my Instagram app in case she responded and saw that I had read the response right away, like I was waiting for it. (Didn't want to seem too enthusiastic.)

Then I got a notification. *Omg she already wrote back!* I read the message.

> Bunny! I'm so glad you reached out. I've been wanting to reach out and see if you wanted to hang out, but I was too nervous lol! Yes, I'd love to get a drink, are you available next week?

I not only felt happy that she wanted to hang, but was also comforted that she too felt nervous to reach out. When we get vulnerable, it can help other people feel comfortable being vulnerable as well.

From the Higher Self perspective, friendships not only provide the emotional support that you deserve, but an acknowledgment that if we want to create a world where everyone is valued, then we need to prioritize connectedness on a deeper level. Having meaningful relationships beyond the romantic and familial helps us remember we have always needed each other, and we always will. Does this mean you have to be friends with everyone you meet? No! But it does mean you recognize you are connected on a very deep level to everyone you meet, and that everyone you meet has value.

Friendship is a beautiful reflection of this truth. It's an expression of care and intimacy not based on a utilitarian purpose. In a culture with so much emphasis on productivity and competition, friendships and community can be a safe space to simply be who you are.

We all have different levels of comfort when it comes to socializing. And that is okay. For some people like me, it's not that easy to talk to someone I don't know at a party. For other people, it is. Understanding that a lot of people have varying degrees of social anxiety helps you have more compassion for yourself and helps you realize that the person you are standing next to at a party might be feeling just as uncomfortable as you.

What our Higher Selves want us to understand is that we are enough, and that we deserve to have joy and connection in our lives. We come from a culture that doesn't teach us how to be in community. But we can teach ourselves. Everyone needs love, care, and support in their lives. Sometimes putting yourself out there and reaching out to someone isn't just for yourself — it's a way of letting someone else know that they matter, too.

Maintaining Friendships

Just like romantic relationships, friendships require care, nurturing, and commitment. They also require communication. Many of the guidelines I put in the previous chapter on romantic partnerships apply just as much to friendships.

A healthy, close friendship involves supporting each other's growth and healing; being dependable and trustworthy; respecting each other's needs and boundaries, even when they don't line up; remembering that each person is bringing their wounds and patterns into the relationship; being accountable for your own stuff; and most of all, communicating when things go awry. People assume that friendship isn't a place where you can talk about when you feel hurt because those types of conversations are for romantic partners. But in order to grow a close, intimate friendship, you have to be willing to share your needs and feelings even if it doesn't feel easy.

Let's say for example your friend has a habit of showing up late when you meet up. *How can they be so inconsiderate?* you think to yourself. But rather than telling them how you feel, you just hold it in, and each time it happens you feel more disrespected. Finally, one day while waiting for them to show up late again, you send them an angry text. *Once again, I'm here waiting for you. Are you even coming?* This makes your friend feel yelled at and talked down to, and by the time they show up they also feel angry and disrespected by you.

Now let's see how connecting to your Higher Self might have prevented the two of you from feeling so disrespected. First, you wouldn't wait so long to communicate with your friend that when they are late it is difficult for you, because you'd know that your needs are valid and that sustaining a loving friendship requires being honest about your needs and feelings. Secondly, you'd recognize that your need for your friend to be on time isn't just about that moment, but also reflects all your past experiences with people who might have hurt you by not being dependable. It could also be triggering one of your LHBs where you fear you aren't worthy of having your needs met. Third, you remember that your friend's inability to show up on time might not have anything to do with you. It could be a habit that the people around them growing up also had, or they really don't do well managing their time. Or maybe they fear disappointing people, so rather than be honest about what they are capable of, they make unrealistic expectations. Either way you understand there is more to the story.

Compassion helps you see through the behavior to the fact that we are all in a different place in our journey of self-acceptance, and in any loving relationship our stuff is eventually going to rub up against our friends' stuff. But it also doesn't mean just accepting any behavior, because your friend might have their reasons. Empowered by your Higher Self, you know it's your right to communicate your feelings, and it doesn't happen through an angry text. It looks more like this: *Hey, I wanted to let you know that I have a difficult time when you show up late and make me wait. I feel anxious when it happens, and it also triggers feelings of not being valued in relationships. Is there something we can do in the future to prevent this? Maybe if you add more time to get ready? Or should I just mentally add*

10 min to whatever time you say you'll be there? I know it's not always easy to manage time.

Communicating through your Higher Self is recognizing the other person's Higher Self as well, which makes whatever you say a lot easier to hear, because it doesn't come with a hierarchical energy of "You are wrong because of this and I am right because of that." Rather, "I know we are different—how can we make this work for both of us?"

Friendship Breakups

Naturally, not all friendships last forever. We change, and often the friendship dynamic is no longer compatible with our authentic growth—and that is okay. It doesn't mean there is something wrong or that the friendship failed. But since our culture doesn't put as much value on platonic relationships as romantic ones, it also doesn't spend much time addressing the heartbreak of a friendship breakup, or even how to break up with a friend. So, when friendships end, there often isn't a lot of closure or outside acknowledgment that losing a friend hurts.

Two months before my wedding, one of my best friends, who was going to be my "person of honor" at the ceremony, ghosted me. To this day, I don't know why she did. I've texted, called, left voicemails crying and begging for an answer, but I've never gotten an explanation.

It was obvious she had her reasons for not wanting or being able to be my friend any longer. But she lacked the ability to communicate them. This way of handling the situation made me feel like she had never truly cared about me. Connecting to my Higher Self helped me realize that people's comfort around communicating difficult decisions, boundaries, or emotions is complex.

It also helped me see that relationships are never just about one person's choices. There were many moments in our friendship where she had flaked out on me, not following through with commitments. But rather than be honest about how that made me feel, I often just tried to forget about it. I was scared to bring up difficult things with her, because I was afraid of losing her. If I was honest about my needs, she might think I was too much. Looking back, I often diminished myself in our friendship.

Your Higher Self uses all your experiences as a curriculum for more self-acceptance and self-worth. Going through that difficult friendship breakup was a lesson for me—that if my needs aren't being met in a friendship, I need to speak up. Even if that means I have to face the difficult truth that the friendship isn't healthy or sustainable. That doesn't mean all my needs are more important than my friend's needs—it means that both of our needs are valid, and that both of us need to be committed to making it work.

Friendships are loving and joyful, and they are also sacred and healing. Aligning with your Higher Self will help you navigate the ups and downs of friendships, understand that your friendship is a divine gift you have to offer, and see that everyone deserves connection.

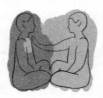

Bring Your Higher Self to Your Friendships

1. **Keep in mind that most people want and need more friends.** I hear it all the time on my podcast, *XO Higher Self*: Listeners telling me that now that they are out of school and dedicated to their careers and/or families, they don't know how to make new friends. And I always remind them that so

many people out there are looking for the same thing. Start by reaching out to acquaintances or people in your periphery you feel interested in getting to know better and actually *try* to be their friend.

Having friends requires putting yourself out there. Send a text or DM and ask to get a cup of coffee, or go on a walk, or maybe have a get-together at your house and invite some new people. Second, get involved in an activity that is social. It can be a dance class or ceramics class or book club. It can be volunteering or community organizing or a spiritual group. Sometimes just doing something that puts you in a social situation is enough to remind yourself how much you like people! Oh, and don't give up if the first thing doesn't work. Keep trying!

2. **Prioritize your friendships even when you are in a committed romantic partnership/and or have a family to take care of.** Besides the benefit of being able to have joyful friendships, having healthy bonds outside your romantic relationship and family helps your family life too! Your partner cannot fulfill all your social needs, and putting that kind of pressure on your partner is not sustainable or healthy. When you connect with friends and have social time outside your family, it helps you remember that your identity is much more than the role you have at home. Spending independent time away from your family helps you appreciate and love them even more.

3. **Tell your friends when something they did hurt your feelings.** Love takes vulnerability. When you are courageous about your feelings, not only is that giving them the respect they deserve, but it also paves the way for your friends to be open about their feelings too. In all our relationships, we have the opportunity to set an example of self-acceptance, compassion, healthy boundaries, and honesty. When we show up aligned in our Higher Selves, we inspire our loved ones to do that as well.

4. **No more frenemies.** Are you in a "friendship" with someone you have a rivalry with and are always trying to outdo? Do you have a "friend" who always puts you down or tries to be competitive, who makes you uncomfortable? Feeling competitive while playing basketball or a game of gin rummy is one thing—but a lot of people hang out together to use each other as punching bags for their insecurities or fears of inadequacy. It's so common that people actually think having frenemies is okay. It's not. Friends do not try to belittle each other.

It's natural to have conflict, say something you don't mean, and be emotionally immature from time to time — no one is perfect. But in your heart, you know the difference between spending time with someone who genuinely wants you to be happy and someone who wants you to feel bad about yourself. If you have a friend who isn't treating you right, speak up. Being open can create the possibility for some needed realizations and deep healing. And if it backfires or your feelings are diminished or ignored, then you know that this is not a healthy friendship and it might be time to walk away.

5. **Express your appreciation to the friends in your life.** A good friend of mine sends me a homemade postcard a couple of times a year just saying hi and that they value our friendship. It's something they do for all their friends, and it makes me feel so special every time I receive one. These little efforts, whether it's sending a card or a text that says, *I just wanted to let you know I am so happy to have you in my life,* go a long way. Not only are these loving things to do for your friends, but they keep you in a place of gratitude for the people in your life.

Journal Prompts

1. Growing up it was difficult/easy/both difficult and easy for me to make friends because...

    _____

2. My first experience in friendship as a child was...

    _____

3. How those experiences have shaped my perspective on friendships now is...

    _____

4. Being a good friend means...

    _____

5. Reasons why I am a good friend are...

    _____

6. Mistakes I've made in my friendships are...

    _____

7. Things I learned from those mistakes are...

    _____

Films That Celebrate Friendship

Okay, this list is kind of corny, I know, but I can't help myself. I'm a sucker for a friendship flick!

Beaches
Anne of Green Gables
Boys on the Side
Now and Then
Stand By Me
The Secret Garden
Land Before Time
Romy and Michele's High School Reunion
Booksmart
Steel Magnolias

Chapter 10

Race and Healing

Me: *We live in a racist world.*
Higher Self: *We live in a world where racism is systemically ingrained in us. We can change that system, and change the world.*

I didn't want to be different.

"In the year 2000, the majority of the population in Dallas will be Hispanic," said my fifth grade teacher, Miss Drumond, during our social studies lesson.

"Then I'm moving out of Dallas!" yelled Aiden, the class clown with bright red hair who reminded me of Ronald McDonald.

The whole class laughed at Aiden's joke. I felt a lump in my throat, terrified that any moment someone was going to look over at me sitting at my desk and say, "Hey, aren't YOU Mexican?" And then the whole class would turn around and stare like I was one of those optical illusion images that once you see you can't unsee.

I put my head down and pretended to take notes. Thankfully, Mrs. Drumond ignored Aiden's comment and continued with the lesson. I breathed a sigh of relief when I realized that no one was looking at me. But just in case, I kept my head down for the rest of class.

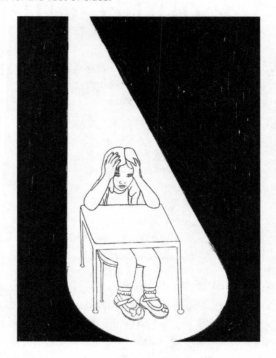

Growing up as a Brown kid in a white suburb of Dallas felt like having a bug bite that gets itchy only if you scratch it. The more I thought about being different from my friends and schoolmates, the more uncomfortable I was—the best way to not feel uncomfortable was to try not to think about it. That's why I hated when anyone pointed it out, like when parents would ask where I was from, or when my fellow students would expect me to know the words in Spanish class, or when my friends said things like, "Wow, your skin is so dark!"

I hated when my dad corrected my pronunciation of Spanish words, especially in front of other people. It didn't help that all of my white friends lived in big houses and that I shared a room with both my sisters in an apartment. (My mom insisted on living in the white neighborhood because it had better schools.)

My favorite TV and movie stars were pretty white girls, like Kelly Kapowski on *Saved by the Bell* and Vada from *My Girl*. I used to wish I had blue eyes like Vada and got excited when I heard of colored contact lenses.

It wasn't that I consciously wanted to be white. I wanted all the things I thought whiteness stood for: prettiness, popularity, money. From my point of view, to be white meant your life was easy. Your parents weren't stressed about paying the bills, and you could look like Shirley Temple or Miss America or one of those angels on the Hallmark cards. (I never saw any pictures of angels with brown skin.)

Another way I tried to blend in was with the pronunciation of my name. My legal name is Melisa. But my first grade teacher pronounced it like Melissa. I was too scared to correct her. And then I noticed I really liked being called Melissa instead of Melisa. Melissa definitely sounded prettier, that is, more white.

The Wounds of Racism

To be on the receiving end of racism, in personal experiences and through systemic racial discrimination, is being forced to ingest a toxic concoction of generational ignorance and hatred. Sometimes you don't see it coming and sometimes you do. It can happen while you are walking down the street, at school, or in your workplace. It can happen while watching a movie, streaming a show, reading the news, or scrolling on social media; it can be the subtle and not-so-subtle barriers to career opportunities, school admittance, or fair treatment at the doctor's office. In a culture organized around racist

LHBs, there is very little social protection from the deep wounds that racism leaves on the psyche and spirit. Is it any surprise how easy it is to struggle with self-worth if you have been made to feel you are inferior? Is it any surprise you might struggle accepting yourself when historically the message you have received was that in certain spaces you are unacceptable?

Experiences of racism literally "get under the skin," explains the trauma expert Gabor Maté. Studies have shown that racial trauma harms people psychologically and physiologically through "the triggering of inflammation-promoting genes, the premature aging of chromosomes and cells, tissue damage, elevation of blood sugar, [and] the narrowing of airways." In other words, racism hurts emotionally, mentally, and physically.

But being the victim of racial discrimination is not an indication that you are not worthy; it is an indication that a toxic culture — based on the falsehood that in order to be good enough you need to be better than other people — is unworthy of you.

Learning Racial Superiority

Racial oppression has existed since ancient civilizations, but the popularization of the idea that racial superiority was a scientific fact began in early modern Europe during the end of the seventeenth century and beginning of the eighteenth century. The historian Siep Stuurman attributes the first racial classification to a French philosopher, physician, and traveler, Francois Bernier, coinciding with France's expansion of colonial slave trade and regulated slavery laws: the Code Noir (1685). His system of classifying mankind, called "Types of Race," was the first to theorize that all people had a race based on their physical features.

Bernier was a pioneer in what would later be a trend of "scientific racism" in Western culture that attempted to categorize human beings into racial hierarchies, justifying the superiority of white Europeans based on biological differences such as brain size, skin color, and body shape. This supposed "evidence" of racial hierarchy reverberated in anthropological, scientific, intellectual, and political thought through the American and French Revolutions.

The United States government has legislated white supremacy throughout its history, including in the drafting of the U.S. Constitution, which protected the institution of slavery; the Removal Act (1830), a violent mass exile of Indigenous peoples from their land; Jim Crow laws intent on disenfranchising Black people and their descendants; and the 1924 Johnson-Reed Act, in which Congress drastically restricted immigration, effectively cutting off all immigration from Asian countries in an attempt to preserve white homogeneity in America. Sadly, the list of laws upholding white supremacy in America is much longer, and racist policies still exist today.

As children, we don't understand how ingrained these beliefs are in the makeup of our shared culture. But that doesn't shield us from their influence. We grow up adopting these biases, believing that we are either superior or inferior (sometimes switching back and forth depending on the context), and they are one of the most detrimental barriers to accessing the love of our Higher Selves, which is our true nature.

I didn't want to be one of them.

On Christmas Eve when I was eleven years old, I sang "Feliz Navidad" in the children's choir at church. I wore a crushed velvet maroon dress, white tights, and black shoes that were so shiny, you could see the lights of the Nativity scene reflecting off them.

In an effort to celebrate "diversity" at our church, the choir leader had the idea to group all the Black and Brown kids together to sing "Feliz Navidad" for the audience, while the white kids' choir got to sing "Rudolph the Red-Nosed Reindeer."

When I found out I was going to have to be part of the "diversity" choir, I was humiliated. Why couldn't I sing with the regular kids? I knew I wasn't white, but at school, all my friends were white. *I don't fit in with the other choir,* I thought. *I don't fit in with...them.*

My reluctance was subdued that week in rehearsal, when I made a new friend, Asha, a pretty Black girl I was assigned to stand next to in the choir. She started talking to me right away; she was in the fourth grade, like me, and she was really nice. For the Christmas Eve service, Asha wore a red and black plaid dress with white lace, and a bow in her hair. I really liked her dress.

Our performance of "Feliz Navidad" went okay. The audience smiled at us a lot, and I almost forgot the embarrassment of not being included in the other choir.

After the applause died down, our group returned to our assigned seats in the pew behind the other kids' choir.

The excitement of having performed on stage made Asha and me giggle the moment we made eye contact after sitting down. Which made Vanessa, from the other choir, turn around in her seat and give Asha and me a look of total disgust. "SHH-HHHH!!!" she hissed.

I had never seen a look like that before, as if we were the grossest things she had ever set eyes on and our giggles were full of cooties. Vanessa and her family were very respected at our church. At Sunday School, she seemed to know all the Bible stories. Unlike me—I only knew about Adam and Eve and Noah's Ark, and a little bit about Moses.

I had talked to Vanessa before, and she had never looked at me that way. But when I was sitting there next to Asha, it was like she saw me as a different person. I was embarrassed and I could feel my throat tighten. I realized I needed to distance myself from my new friend Asha. So, when she tapped my leg trying to get my attention a few minutes later, I kept my eyes focused forward on the manger on stage, with the blond, blue-eyed baby Jesus inside.

As a child, the only way for me to escape the self-loathing of being Brown was to distance myself from my own heritage and to distance myself from associating with the "other." The other could be other Brown kids, Black kids, Asian kids—anyone who, by association, might make me less palatable to whiteness.

I wanted to fit in, to be accepted, and to be liked. The racism and colorism I was being conditioned with made me believe that the darker your skin was, the less valuable you were. When I was with white kids and nobody said anything about me being Brown, I could almost forget I wasn't white. But when I was around Brown and Black kids, it was in my face, unavoidable, like holding up a mirror to the parts of myself that made me inferior.

―――――――――

You Are Not Your Conditioning

We all come from a shared history of white supremacy and colorism. The idea that centuries of these societal beliefs would not affect how we see ourselves and each other today is unrealistic. Many of those beliefs operate unconsciously, in quick judgments, biases, and denials of injustice. Many of those beliefs manifest as low self-worth, emotional suppression, and/or denying your needs.

The process of connecting to your Higher Self requires bringing your Learned Hierarchical Beliefs into your awareness. But it doesn't stop there. It also means understanding that **your conditioning isn't who you are.** That way you can replace those learned beliefs with loving truths.

Looking at your racial wounds and/or your unconscious racial bias isn't an easy process. For many of you there is no way to "not see" racism because you yourself experience it. However, we often don't connect our racial wounds with our internalized low self-worth. LHBs are designed for you to take all the blame for feeling bad about yourself. They make you feel there is something wrong with you and then make you feel there is something wrong with you for feeling that way. The process of healing racial wounds begins with acknowledging that as much as you don't believe in the validity of white supremacy, it is still very much part of the equation when you're stuck in fears of inadequacy or self-loathing thoughts.

Likewise, many white people would say that white supremacy is bad while at the same time being unwilling to engage with ways it shapes their beliefs, thoughts, and behaviors.

It's easy to get defensive when someone points out your privilege or racial bias if you don't understand where your conditioning comes from. It's easy to be paralyzed in guilt if you think what you have been taught to believe makes you an inherently bad person. But people are not inherently bad—they've been misguided. **The reason it is so hard for some people to let go of their own privilege is because they don't know their value without it.** Who am I if I'm not better than those other people? And anything that in their mind threatens that privilege becomes a threat to their way of life.

Looking back at my childhood experience in the church choir is painful on multiple levels: first that I was on the receiving end of racism but even more so that I was a perpetuator of racism— all before I even truly understood what racism was. I can both have compassion for myself because I was raised in a socially racist environment and acknowledge how harmful and toxic my behavior was.

Connecting to my Higher Self helped me see the ways I benefit in a white supremacist system because I know that my conditioning isn't my true nature. And in order to keep unlearning, I have to first see the insidious ways that conditioning influences my perspective.

Learned Hierarchical Beliefs are harmful to everyone, no matter where you are on the ladder of that racial hierarchy. Any belief that tells you your worth is determined by the color of your skin is a barrier to knowing true self-worth.

Confronting my wounds

My white girlfriend broke up with me for calling her racist. Okay, it's a little more complicated than that. In the years leading up to our breakup in 2015, there had been a smattering of news stories about police killing Black people: Trayvon Martin, Michael Brown, Eric Garner, Tamir Rice...The Black Lives Matter movement had spurred new conversations in mainstream culture, especially on social media, about white supremacy: how prevalent white violence is in this country, and the many forms that racism takes.

The concept of white privilege was entering mainstream consciousness. When I was young, either you were racist or you weren't, and being racist meant you were in the KKK, had a Confederate flag sticker on your car, or were one of those neo-Nazis on *The Ricki Lake Show*. I didn't understand that the comments kids made about my skin were rooted in white supremacy—that racism is social conditioning that infiltrates our culture to greater and lesser degrees. I just thought they knew something I didn't. And I never really addressed those wounds, or fully understood how those experiences shaped my self-perception.

The Black Lives Matter movement and online discourse on white supremacy and privilege opened up a new awareness within me and also helped me to see my own privilege and conditioned racism as a non-Black person of color. I wanted to be more accountable, and I also wanted to be part of the solution. What I didn't realize was that in order to do that, I had to address my own pain.

It amazes me how much has changed in our collective consciousness since 2015. Most so-called progressive liberal queer white people that I hung around with at that time were not willing to say they benefited from white privilege. In fact, they excused insensitive behavior. This is where my relationship with my partner started to break down.

On multiple occasions, when I would call out comments that people in our circle made as rooted in white privilege, my girlfriend at the time would defend their behavior rather than validate my perspective, as if she knew what constituted racism better than I did.

I was so raw with emotion and unaddressed wounds that the only recourse I had at the time was rage and anger. This only reinforced her belief that I was the one with the problem.

My "anger issues" became a narrative in our relationship that I resented. And I carried that resentment into other areas of our relationship as well. I became resentful of paying half of our rent and bills when she made more money than I did. I resented her rich white friends, and her choice of a career in commercial real estate, which I saw as a modern form of colonialism. These resentments came out in alcohol-fueled tantrums that pushed us further and further apart. It all culminated in one last fight, in which I told her that it wasn't just that she benefited from white privilege, but that she herself was racist. It was the last straw for her. She said it was over.

Her inability to validate my pain and the subsequent abandonment of the relationship was like a knife in the wound. It seemed to say, *See, you aren't good enough for white people, and you never will be.*

Becoming aware of how racism has caused harm in your personal life and in our collective is a painful process of disillusionment. Anger and rage are necessary in the process of healing. Those emotions are indications of wounds that deserve to be acknowledged. Not only do we have a lack of education about how racism, white supremacy, and colorism are still causing harm in our society, but we also lack a support system for our healing and unlearning. We need more safe spaces where our anger and rage can be expressed. We need more education on how we got here.

What I needed in 2015 was the support of people who understood what I was going through. And my ex-girlfriend was not that person. It wasn't until I was able to speak to a therapist that I began to understand that there was nothing wrong with my anger. The silencing of pain and suffering only perpetuates oppression. I was no longer that little kid in school who kept their head down out of fear that my presence might take the fun out of their racist jokes.

Both my ex-girlfriend and myself were ill-equipped to handle the awakening that was happening inside me, her inability or unwillingness to see how much her white privilege needed to be addressed, and the resulting shift in our relationship. Because I had never dealt with my own wounds, her dismissiveness felt like a dismissal of my entire past experience.

I know that isn't what she intended to do. I know that she didn't realize the power she had over me in those moments. She didn't know that what I needed was healing—and honestly, neither did I at the time. My anger and emotions were especially difficult for her because she came from a difficult family situation. So she often reverted to walling up and avoiding confrontation as a way to feel safe.

Connecting to my Higher Self and seeing the Higher Self in my ex helped me realize that it wasn't that I was unlovable—it was that she didn't know how to love me, and in those moments, I also didn't know how to love myself. Although we are no longer in contact, I know our shared experience helped both of us grow in ways we didn't realize we needed.

Compassion as Self Preservation

Compassion is a source of power when you are confronting racism. Compassion doesn't mean accepting other people's insensitive, harmful, or hateful behavior; it's understanding that behind that behavior lie unaddressed wounds and internalized fears of inadequacy, perpetuated by a racist belief system. A person's ability or inability to come to terms with that reflects where they are in the journey of self-awareness—not your own value or worthiness. Compassion is the vision to see beyond the behavior, thus empowering yourself in the face of their attempts at projection.

If we want to dismantle the destructive, abusive, and toxic impacts of racism, we have to look at the causal level and not focus only on the effects. Similar to healing disease in the body, we not only have to address the symptoms—that is, the harmful behavior of racist people—but we also have to look at the belief system that enables racism to metastasize. That deeper understanding will empower our fight against racism, because it helps us heal our own wounds. Again, we often don't make the connection between our racial trauma and how it manifests as low self-worth. Compassion is the vision that separates who we are from our LHBs. So the next time we are stuck in a bout of self-loathing thoughts, we can ask ourselves, *Who put this voice into my head? Is it my Higher Self—the part of me that knows I am whole and enough just for being me? Or is this a voice of white supremacy?*

To be clear, this does not mean it's your responsibility to heal the people who are harming you, or to continue to give your time and energy to them if it would better serve you to set boundaries. But it is your responsibility to heal yourself, and that cannot happen if you are stuck in the same hierarchical mindset of superior versus inferior.

Contrary to popular belief, calling out someone's harmful behavior *is* an act of compassion and comes from love. This is not love in the sense of needing to love someone who is denying your humanity. Coming from love means honoring your inner awareness that love is true power—a power that all of us are individually responsible for awakening within ourselves.

Show Up with Your Higher Self

Your Higher Self can help you unlearn racist LHBs as a white or non-BIPOC and become part of our collective healing. The first thing is acknowledging that you have picked up these biases to a greater and lesser degree living in a racist society and you have benefited from a hierarchical system that assigns you value based on your race. But that doesn't mean you are a bad person or that you aren't enough. You are not defined by the LHBs you are unlearning. Connecting to that truth will empower you. Shaming yourself for your own privilege keeps you in the same low self-worth that makes you vulnerable to LHBs. You didn't create a racist system. But you do have a responsibility to help dismantle it. Seeing through the lens of your Higher Self will inspire you to educate yourself, to listen when people are talking about their experiences of racism, to have compassion for how painful and difficult it is to be a victim of racism, and to stand up for our shared humanity in the face of racism in your personal life and on a collective level by advocating for changes in laws and policies. Your Higher Self can help you sustain your inner and outer work and do it with love and encouragement because you recognize that everyone (including you) deserves love, care, and to live in a society that values them.

I know I am not finished with my inner work and the healing of my own racist conditioning. As a non-Black person of color who has also experienced racism, it's tempting to get defensive when being called out for my own privilege. But I know that defensiveness is a call to ask myself, "What is it that I am defending?" Acknowledging the suffering of others does not negate your own suffering. Acknowledging that you have benefited from white privilege does not mean you haven't struggled in your life.

It's Okay to Not Be Okay

A couple of months ago, Khara and I were at a party at one of our neighbors' houses. One of our new neighbor friends, Greg, mentioned in a group conversation that he bought his house from an older man named Harold, who lived in the house down the road from mine. I had seen Harold watering his yard but had never spoken to him. Greg casually mentioned that Harold had made a comment to him that was a bit off-handedly racist but also said he was a very nice old man. Intuitively I felt the racist comment was about Mexican people, judging by the way Greg, after glancing over at me, seemed to have second thoughts about getting into too much detail. So I pressed him.

"What was the racist thing he said?" I asked.

"Oh, just something dumb about Mexican workers," Greg replied. "I think he is a nice guy, though. He's just old."

For the rest of the party I couldn't think about anything else. How this sweet old guy Harold, who everyone liked, didn't like Mexicans like me, but it didn't seem to do much to change anyone's opinion of him.

When Khara and I got home from the party I told them what happened and started to cry. I was overwhelmed and exhausted—from being the only nonwhite person in that conversation, from having to decide what I would say or not say, from imagining all the racist comments that happened when I was out of earshot. It took me back to all the other experiences I'd had that were painful. I was also worried about running into this Harold guy when I was walking my dog. If I did, what would I say? Are these new neighbors really my friends? Khara just held me and listened. It was all they could do. Since Khara is white and couldn't fully understand the pain I was experiencing, validating my pain by just holding me rather than trying to fix it created a safe space for me to move through it.

We Can Do This with Love

Navigating our racial healing, no matter what your experience has been, is going to be a lifelong practice and process. Some days are going to be harder than others. Sometimes, we will have the energy to confront it, and some days we will be too emotionally overwhelmed and exhausted. But our Higher Selves are here for us, reminding us that every one of us is valuable and worth the effort. There is so much love within all of us. We are not our LHBs. This we must never forget.

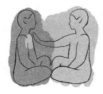

Your Higher Self in Racial Healing

1. **You are not your conditioning.** Whether you were told you are inferior or superior, whether you have let go of those beliefs or they are still a part of your daily experience, your LHBs are not who you really are. Yes, they have impacted your life; but the less you identify with them, the less power they will have over you. You are not a bad person. You are a loving person. You are a beautiful person.

2. **Compassion is your power.** Shaming yourself for the conditioning you are still unlearning or for how your wounds show up in your everyday life only keeps you imprisoned in the same low self-worth that you are trying to heal from and unlearn. Your Higher Self is a voice of compassion and encouragement. It's like a warm hug that lets you know you are safe and whole. Whatever issues you are working through do not make you any less lovable.

3. **It's okay to be angry.** It's like that cliché "The only way out is through." Anger is not a bad emotion. But when you don't let yourself get angry or upset and push that stuff down, it has

nowhere to go and cannot be released. Does that mean you have to start throwing dishes across the room when you get triggered? No, not necessarily. It just means acknowledging, "Okay, I am angry right now. And I have a right to feel that way. How can I give myself grace through this?"

4. **Whites and non-BIPOCs — you're gonna get things wrong.** If you are working on unlearning your LHBs and becoming aware of how your privilege colors your perspective, that is great! But that doesn't mean you won't ever make a mistake. That doesn't mean you won't say or do something that you weren't aware was hurtful to another person ever again. Take those missteps as opportunities to grow. Be open to hearing criticism. Be receptive to learning about other peoples' experiences, and recognize the role your LHBs have played in your own understanding of race and racism. Ask your BIPOC friends how you can best support them. It's not easy, but the more humble you are about your mistakes, the easier it will be to improve and move forward.

5. **Take breaks from news stories and social media when you are feeling overwhelmed. Although "taking a break" from racism IRL is not an option for people who experience it, social media is a place where you do have *some* control over what you are seeing.** There are videos of instances of racism all over TikTok. It seems like every day another act of racism caught on police body cams is playing on the local news. It's important to stay informed, but watching instances of racial abuse and violence can retraumatize you. Be mindful of when you are overwhelmed with emotion and your heart is telling you, *No, not today.* Self-care, rest, and recuperation are vital to continue on your healing path. So trust when you feel it's just too much to take in at the moment. It doesn't mean you don't care.

Affirmations for Healing Racial Wounds

- I honor my ancestors by giving myself the love and compassion I need.
- I am not alone in my experience.
- I surrender my attachment to those who have harmed me.
- The greatest privilege is the privilege to love.
- I believe in humanity's capacity to heal.

Journal Prompts

1. My experiences with racism growing up were...

2. The beliefs I carry about myself and others from those experiences are...

3. Flip the script: My Higher Self would respond to those beliefs with...

4. I deserve compassion for my difficult experiences/I should show compassion to others who have experienced difficulty because...

5. My hopes for the healing of racial wounds in our world are...

6. Active ways I can contribute to our collective racial healing are...

Chapter 11

Politics and Activism

Me: *Why should I believe humanity can ever change?*
Higher Self: *Because you have.*

Us and them

A few months after the 2016 presidential election, I found myself at a dinner party at a friend's parents' house, sitting at a large table of upper-class, highly educated white liberals. The political situation was on everyone's minds, and there was a lot of conversation. Everyone was going around the table talking about how awful, racist, and ignorant Republicans are. It was a dialogue that I had heard and participated in often prior to this evening.

At the time, both my parents were registered Republicans, and I hadn't yet asked them how they voted in the 2016 election.

I was afraid to. I'd already had political arguments with them in the past. I'd already gotten upset, asked how they could have voted for Bush with a gay child. But my dad, a proud Mexican American with a master's degree in political science, has this way of rationalizing everything. He never raises his voice, just calmly explains his reasoning and emphasizes that the Democrats are not helping Hispanics, highlighting his account of how when he worked for the U.S. Hispanic Chamber of Commerce, the Carter administration shut the door on them.

As these rich liberals sipped their expensive wine, I thought about how hard my parents worked and how we never had anything close to what these people had in terms of wealth. How the wealth my fellow diners lived on could probably be traced back to slavery. How we were eating dinner on stolen Lenape land. How European white elitism had created this hierarchy of civilized versus uncivilized, of educated versus ignorant, and how that cycle persists.

I started to feel more and more uncomfortable with the tone of the conversation. It angered me to think people were calling my parents ignorant.

"My parents are Republican," I blurted out. The room got quiet.

"How can your dad be a Republican—isn't he Mexican?" someone said.

"I guess it's more complex than that," I replied.

I realized I had been dissociating from the fact that my parents, two people who I knew loved me and were good people, were also the Republicans whom I had been talking so badly about and blaming for the problems in our country. This dinner party was bringing all of that to the surface. And now I couldn't look away. If my parents were loving and intelligent people who still voted differently from me, that meant there were other loving and intelligent people on the other side.

I left that dinner with a pit in my stomach. I saw clearly that our collective political dilemma was more complex than some people being on the wrong side and some people being on the right side. Blaming the other side was pulling the cover over a deeper understanding. It was dehumanizing the people you complained were behaving in an inhumane way. An us-versus-them mentality was a way to feel more comfortable with who you were without questioning how you might be contributing to the problem.

In the years since, most of us would say that political discourse has gotten worse. The way politics are approached in this country seems almost entirely based around Learned Hierarchical Beliefs. Unchecked capitalism is a breeding ground for greed and corruption in our political system because it prioritizes profit over people. Corporations line the pockets of politicians who are more interested in power than leadership and are willing to create as much divisiveness as necessary to hold on to that power by exploiting our fears and conditioned biases. LHBs are always about "the other," because LHBs say that you are not good enough unless you are better than other people. So you need an "other" to be better than. We see this on display in our politics every day: *My side is better than your side. You are a horrible person because you don't agree with me. You don't deserve the same rights as me because you are a lesser human being.* Politicians use the illusion of the other as a scapegoat for their constituents' struggles. They come into power by promising to destroy this "enemy," often instead of acknowledging their own flaws or a flawed system that is meant to serve only a select few. This is a strategy that has been implemented time and time again, but more often than not it's a distraction from actual solutions and systemic change. It keeps us focused on blaming each other rather than asking how we can make things work for all of us. It keeps us dehumanizing one another rather than seeking leadership that speaks and acts on behalf of our shared humanity. It keeps us in a constant state of trying to win culture wars without asking ourselves, *What is it going to take to cultivate peace in our culture?* As long as our focus is on putting other people down, how can we possibly lift each other up?

Love Is a Political Act

When you think of politics, what are some images that come to mind? Old white men vying for power? Members of House and Senate gridlocked in disagreement, unable to pass legislation? Election drama? Accusations of lying and fraud? Social media spats? Probably the last thing you think of is love. But from the Higher Self perspective, you cannot separate politics from love. Love is a political act.

Choosing love in politics means taking action on behalf of everyone's inherent value, whether that is through your voice, your vote, your organizing, your art, your leadership, or whatever means your heart is calling you toward. Choosing love in politics is refusing to buy into the game of dehumanizing people you don't agree with; it's calling out injustice and lovelessness in our policies and leadership. Choosing love in politics is valuing community over competition and coming together to dismantle the overzealous individualism that has harmed our political system. It's through the empowerment of love that we say, *There is another way.*

Affirming our shared value has to be at the heart of our politics in order to create the peace and equanimity that so many of us deserve and crave. When we let our LHBs color our perspective, we lose sight of the fact that our value doesn't come from having more or being better, but it is inherent to who we all are. In other words, until you see that truth about other people, you won't see it about yourself. We are not separate. We rise and we fall together. As the civil rights leader Fannie Lou Hamer so eloquently put it, "No one is free until everyone is free."

Now, you might say to yourself, *Okay, I agree that everyone has value, but what about the people who support politicians advocating for sexist, homophobic, and racist policies? They are perpetuating harm. So why should I value them?*

There is a difference between loveless behavior and the belief that the people who engage in that behavior are inherently bad people. If we are unable to separate the LHBs from the individual, it makes sense that we would struggle to see the humanity in them, possibly even hate them. It makes sense that the only solution seems like insulting them into changing.

The thing is, people who struggle with having compassion for others are unaware of their true value. They believe that in order to be worthy, they need to villainize and demonize their fellow human beings. They are terrified of not being enough. And so they try to make other people, those who are different from them, not good enough. They have been misguided to believe this is their only form of empowerment. Politics is an arena where their LHBs are easily exploited. Encouraged by power-hungry politicians to focus their grievances on people who are different from them, they find community in those who affirm their hierarchical worldview. Their LHBs become part of their identity, making them feel like they are defending themselves when they defend hateful beliefs. This is learned behavior. They were not born this way.

Seeing this through the lens of your Higher Self won't make you complacent or accepting of harmful behavior and loveless political policies; it will give you the vision to know what is at the heart of the matter. In other words, the perspective that the people who are causing harm aren't as worthy as you exacerbates the problem and keeps the cycle of "othering" going because you are stuck in the same hierarchical mindset. LHBs are so sneaky! You cannot dismantle LHBs and the harm they cause by attaching to your own. We have to tear down the whole system internally; otherwise you will keep playing their hierarchical political game, a game no one wins.

It's important to understand, however, that separating a person's humanity from the LHBs they are conditioned with does not mean you shouldn't call out their destructive behavior and stand vehemently against the harm they are causing. All too often people stay silent in the face of suffering under the guise of "peace and love." As if there is anything loving about witnessing the harm caused by racist, sexist, homophobic, and transphobic policies and turning a blind eye. Love says "no" in the face of loveless behavior. Love protects those who need it. Love gives a voice to those who aren't heard. Our Higher Selves give us the vision to see the LHBs that are motivating people's behavior, and empower us to be representatives of love in the spaces where love is needed. And in many cases that means us taking on the responsibility to say, "Not on my watch!"

It's Going to Take Our Higher Selves

I'm not here to tell you that I have the answers to the profound problems we face today—climate change, poverty, mass incarceration, systemic racism, voter suppression...the list goes on and on. But what I do know is that in order to find solutions, we have to dismantle the hierarchical belief system that allowed these problems to arise and proliferate. We have to put love first by affirming each other's value and defending each other's right to live peaceful, safe, and abundant lives no matter who you are. **The only way to empower humanity is to empower *everyone*.** It's going to take seeing our Higher Selves and the Higher Self in each other. Albert Einstein said, "No problem can be solved from the same level of consciousness it was created." We have to change the consciousness—that is, the belief system—in which we approach our politics. Otherwise we will continue to destroy our planet and each other. There is no other way.

We all carry LHBs. And yet so many of us have found the strength and awareness within us to begin changing and unlearning. If it is possible for you, it is possible for everyone. Truly seeing yourself—that you were created whole, that you are worthy of care, abundance, and safety simply for being you—enables you to see that same truth in others. As Eckhart Tolle says, "To love is to recognize yourself in another."

Activism and Taking Care of Yourself

With so many political issues to address, who wouldn't feel overwhelmed? With war and oppression on a global scale, who wouldn't struggle with balancing their activism and preventing emotional and/or physical burnout? With so many people online chastising each other on the "right" way to speak on an issue, who wouldn't feel fearful or even paralyzed in speaking out, or questioning whether their voice even matters? So how do we contribute to the change we want to see in the world while keeping ourselves safe and tending to our own well-being?

Political activism from the Higher Self perspective is about staying conscious as to what is motivating you. Is it your LHBs that will use anything including your political activism as a way to feel not good enough, or is it your Higher Self that knows you have always been good enough and activism is about calling out injustice and empowering all people, including yourself?

It's all too common that people who are consistently showing up to help others, who courageously stand up against oppression in their activism, deny themselves rest and recuperation— sometimes even guilting themselves for having the relative safety and privilege to be able to care for their basic needs. LHBs are the inner oppressor that will mask self-destructive patterns as virtue and self-improvement. Dismantling oppression is an external and internal journey. No matter who you are, addressing the suffering in the world takes a toll on you mentally, emotionally, spiritually, and sometimes physically, because stress can have physiological effects in the body. Self-care is absolutely necessary.

On the other side of the spectrum, the shame of "not being enough" brought on by a culture that teaches people they are inherently lacking can manifest as cynicism, lack of empathy, dissociation and denial, and feeling paralyzed into inaction when it comes to helping others or speaking out against injustice. Many people struggle with understanding how important they are and how powerful their love is. Feelings of guilt can be a catalyst for someone to see the harmful effects of their inaction, however, in my experience it usually results in a temporary change or what some people label "performative virtue signaling," possibly resulting in a post on social media and going no further. Sustainable activism comes from the realization that everyone is needed in awakening love on the planet. Your perspective and experience are valuable because you belong here. If you have been hesitant, I want you to think about what put that voice in your head that tells you you don't have anything to give or that your participation doesn't make a difference. Or that "nothing will ever change, so what's the point." Can you hear how disempowering that is? That is the voice of an oppressive belief system you have been conditioned with. It's time to break free.

No matter where you are on the spectrum of your activism, it's important to understand that it isn't going to feel *comfortable*. Because activism is challenging the status quo, or what you are used to. You will have to push yourself, but the form that it takes depends on where you can more fully show up for love in your own life and in others'. Sometimes that will mean learning from mistakes, being more compassionate to yourself, having difficult conversations, not avoiding confrontations, being accountable in ways you didn't anticipate, or even losing social media followers (hello, wellness influencers who stay silent in the face of global suffering!), but what could be more important than waking up to the power of our Higher Selves that knows we are here to awaken more love on the planet?

Activism from the Higher Self perspective means realizing that caring for humanity and caring for yourself go hand in hand. There are so many ways to contribute, but the form of that contribution is less important than the consciousness you bring to it. Staying aligned and embodied in your Higher Self is the grounding you need to keep your activism sustainable and to remember why you are doing it: to put more love into the world.

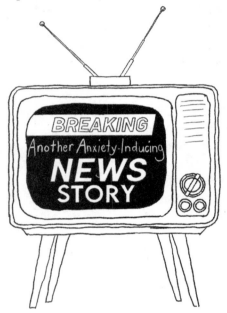

Holding on to Hope

When you are reading the news and the opinion pieces about why this politician is horrible and why the country is on the brink of destruction, it can feel like there is no reason to hope things will change. But it's important to remember that most of what we read in the news or that gets shared on social media is focused on pointing out people's wrongs and not people's rights. Our cultural LHBs have us so driven to judge and criticize each other that the loudest voices of judgment and criticism are the ones that get amplified. The people who say the most offensive and hurtful things get the highest TV ratings, have the most popular political podcasts, and sell the most newspapers. Hope and optimism do not sell the way cynicism, hatred, and negativity do. And so we get a distorted representation of how most people feel. Most people want to live peaceful, joyful, abundant lives with their loved ones.

When I am feeling bogged down in hopelessness about the state of the world, I like to think about all the moments of love I see every day—the kind smile from the barista at the coffee shop, the stranger who insists I go first at a stop sign, the mom hugging and kissing her toddler at the grocery store, the elderly man who told me to have a beautiful day when we passed each other walking our dogs...This is who we really are. There are innumerable acts of love and compassion in the world every day—far more than acts of hatred and lovelessness. There are countless activists both in history and today who stand up for their fellow human beings in the face of countless obstacles. Every positive political change toward a more equal and just society began with people believing we can do this another way. This truth is where I source my hope from. Seeing the Higher Selves in each other is a decision to expand your perception to see who people are beyond their LHBs. If we leave it up to the media or popular culture to give us that perspective, we miss out on so much love.

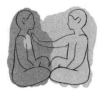

Bring Your Higher Self to Politics and Activism

1. **Boundaries, boundaries, boundaries!** You cannot help others if you are not taking care of yourself. Doing things like reading the news before you go to bed or getting into an argument with a stranger on social media about white supremacy might not be the best strategies for keeping your activism and political participation healthy and sustainable. Inner peace and presence keep you connected to the wisdom of your Higher Self, who knows which choices are helpful and which are harmful. Just as all your relationships need boundaries to be healthy, so does your relationship to politics and activism.

2. **Don't shame yourself for not understanding how our political system functions.** A lot of people shy away from politics because they feel intimidated. How do taxes work? Who is my local congressperson? What is the Electoral College? It's okay! Many people in power prefer their constituents to be politically ignorant so they won't try to change anything. It's never too late to educate yourself about politics. It will empower you to know what your tax money is paying for or how your vote will affect your life. Your perspective, needs, and voice matter! Who knows where some more understanding might lead? (Maybe . . . running for office yourself?)

3. **Don't shame people for being disheartened by politics and feeling unmotivated to participate.** When you feel like your government has never worked in your best interests or has deliberately oppressed you, it's totally understandable to be

cynical and pessimistic that voting or participating in politics will ever make a difference. When generations upon generations of people in your community are constantly disappointed in the lack of progress on their basic human rights, it's easy to throw in the towel. In the aftermath of the 2016 election, there was a lot of blaming those who didn't vote — but the issue is much more complex than that. The truth is, people have been continually disenfranchised by our political system. To blame the outcome of an election on those people is off the mark. What we need to do is recognize that their feelings and experiences are often things we have never gone through and should not judge. Instead, we should listen to their perspective while affirming that their voice matters. Focus on uplifting people by giving them the respect they are entitled to.

4. **Stop demonizing the other side.** When you stop seeing the humanity in other people, it disempowers you. You lose sight of the fact that bigotry and hatred are taught. You stop being able to distinguish between fighting against hatred and wanting to destroy the people who have been conditioned to hate. Hatred is a sickness. The only way to heal it is to stop fueling it by hating in response. That doesn't mean you don't speak up when someone is causing harm — it means you counter that hatred with wisdom and love.

5. **You don't have to have an opinion about something you don't fully understand.** There is this need in social media to have an opinion or a hot take on everything political or controversial. And a lot of people, afraid of being on the "wrong" side of the argument, jump on the bandwagon without fully comprehending a situation that is often more complex than a social media post can illustrate. It's okay to be unsure of how you think about something.

6. **Everyone's activism can look different.** For some people, attending a protest is an overwhelming and overstimulating experience. Some people would rather keep their political

opinions off the internet. For others, their activism looks like giving voice to anger because their anger has been silenced—and aggressive language is exactly the tone that inspires them. Taking a calmer, studied approach to an issue helps others process it without emotional burnout. There isn't one right way to inspire change, because we all come from different experiences and have different relationships to language. If something isn't for you, that doesn't mean it's wrong or bad, it's just not for you. Find leaders, community, and ways to participate that help you sustain your journey, keep you inspired, and make you feel empowered.

Affirmations

- I believe in the capacity for humanity to heal.
- I am a gift to this world.
- I can't care for others without caring for myself.
- Being overwhelmed with the world does not mean there is something wrong with me. It means I am a compassionate person who cares. My tender heart is beautiful.

Journal Prompts

1. When I think about politics I feel . . .

2. Possible ways I can become more politically active are . . .

3. Boundaries and/or changes in my behavior to have a healthier relationship to politics and activism are . . .

4. What would your Higher Self say about people who disagree with you politically?

_____

5. Ways I can be a representative of love when it comes to politics are...

_____

6. I am worthy of living in a safe and peaceful world because...

_____

Chapter 12

Beauty and Body Image

Me: *I look in the mirror and I don't like what I see.*
Higher Self: *That's because you are not really seeing*
yourself; you're seeing how close or far away you
are from a standard of beauty you have been
conditioned to believe in.

Looking good and feeling bad

My first real relationship with exercise began in 2009, when my roommate convinced me to go to a hot yoga class. It was one of the most challenging physical experiences I'd had to date, but my natural flexibility gave me a boost of confidence. Finally I had found something "athletic" that I wasn't the worst at. I loved it. I went back two days later without my roommate, and kept going.

My initial goal for yoga was to be healthier, and I was surprised at the several pounds I dropped from practicing for just a few months. At the time, I understood the cultural pressure to be skinny came from sexist body ideals. I was fully aware that the modeling and fashion industry put unrealistic expectations on us. When a magazine quoted the supermodel Kate Moss saying, "Nothing tastes as good as skinny feels" (which she now deeply regrets saying), I cringed at the thought of people taking that advice. So when my weight kept dropping, I told myself, *This isn't about being skinny, this is about being healthy.* I'd look at myself in the mirror and smile at my progress, promising myself I would keep going. I loved my new body and it seemed like other people did too. When I'd run into someone I hadn't seen for a while they would comment, "Wow, you look great!" I figured the fitter I got, the happier I would be. I began practicing six days a week. If I missed a class, I would feel guilty. If my poses weren't improving, I felt like I

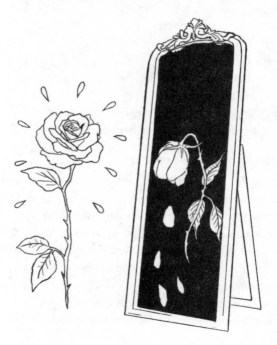

wasn't trying hard enough. I started to become more and more anxious about how I looked. I'd check the scale constantly. I'd berate myself for eating dessert. Eventually, looking in the mirror didn't feel good because I was constantly measuring my progress. If I didn't see "improvement," I'd panic. The initial boost of confidence that losing weight gave me turned into fear. I was terrified of going back to the weight I was before — although ironically, when I was that weight I wasn't as unhappy as I was becoming. I told myself that yoga was making me healthier and happier, but looking back, I question how healthy I really was if the thought of gaining any weight had the power to make me feel worthless.

Beauty Standards: More Than Skin Deep

Over the last five years or so, openly discussing the harmful effects of beauty standards has become mainstream. We see more diverse body shapes in fashion advertisements, TV shows, and movies. Body positivity is trending on social media. But for so many of us, despite increasing awareness of how damaging beauty standards can be — that they have been largely shaped by the cis white male gaze — when we look in the mirror, it's difficult to translate that understanding to our own bodies. We either feel shame about how our body looks or shame because we still don't like how we look even though there is more "representation" and we are aware beauty standards are harmful. And yes, it absolutely helps to see more people who look like you be included in what our culture says is beautiful.

But beauty standards have always been about so much more than mere aesthetics — they have been a measurement of inner worth. LHB-fueled beauty standards such as fatphobia, ableism, and colorism have been historically used not just to quantify physical attraction but also as indicators of intelligence, moral standing, mental pathology, sexual deviance, and a measurement of the value of a human being within a community. This is quite literally more than skin-deep.

And that is why changing how we look, or the appearance of our beauty icons, does not automatically change how we see ourselves. When we don't know our inherent value, we won't see it in the mirror.

In *Fearing the Black Body: The Racial Origins of Fat Phobia*, Sabrina Strings illustrates the historical shift from equating fatness with beauty to racializing fatness as a so-called biological marker of inferiority. During the Renaissance, male European artists and philosophers studied the scholars of ancient Rome and Greece in an attempt to ascertain which physical qualities exemplify true beauty. Artistic works celebrated full-bodied, curvaceous white women with "pointed noses and fine lips" — facial features associated with European descent. However, as the Atlantic slave trade expanded, so did the need to differentiate white bodies from racial "others" to support the narrative of European/Anglo-Saxon superiority. Strings explains that racial scientific discourse during the Enlightenment linked body size to racial category and "transformed the act of eating from personal to political."

It wasn't just body size and color under scrutiny. After the 1871 publication of Charles Darwin's *Descent of Man*, which linked body hair to the evolutionary shift between "man" and "brute," attitudes toward body hair began to change in American culture. As Rebecca M. Herzig explains in her book *Plucked: A History of Hair Removal*, "differences in hair type and amount came to be described as effects of evolutionary forces. The pathologizing of 'excessive' hair growth... by the dawn of the twentieth century, had established [hairiness] as a sign of sexual, mental, and criminal deviance."

The beauty hierarchy would become more firmly established in the United States with the influx of immigration. Anti-immigration propaganda used caricatures to emphasize physical features that existed outside that "normative" framework as a threat to society. The eugenics movement arose in the first half of the twentieth century in the United States, influenced by a distorted interpretation of social Darwinism and natural selection. Eugenicists believed that what they saw as ideal physical characteristics were a product of a higher evolutionary state, and that immigration and the mixing of races was degrading the Anglo-Saxon superior race. People with physical disabilities, along with many other marginalized groups, were deemed unfit for reproduction. From 1907 to 1963, 64,000 individuals were forcibly sterilized as a result of eugenics legislation in the United States.

The expansion of mass media and popular culture in the first half of the twentieth century enabled the proliferation of racist, sexist, and ableist beauty ideals. Advertisements for emotionally and physically toxic beauty products popped up in newspapers and magazines, including advertisements for edible arsenic wafers that supposedly made your skin paler but were also deadly, radioactive creams and toothpaste, pills containing tapeworms for weight loss, and thallium hair removal treatments.

Measuring up to LHBs about beauty standards was about much more than *looking* good—it was about *being* good enough. Someone who was convinced they needed to fit into that ideal became a target consumer for the expanding beauty industry as well as the health and wellness industry.

Diet Culture

We have long been told that skinny equals healthy and fat equals unhealthy. But it is that belief that has put so many people's health at risk. In her book *Anti-Diet,* Christy Harrison argues that the "obesity epidemic" is largely manufactured. When the National Institutes of Health (NIH), a U.S. federal agency, claimed that one third of the U.S. population was overweight in 1995, and then set the American standards for body mass index (BMI) in 1998, millions of Americans were instantaneously put into the category of obese. The NIH's findings were based on a report by the World Health Organization, which based its report on a study conducted by the International Obesity Task Force—a study funded by pharmaceutical companies selling weight-loss drugs.

The consequences of these reports were that many millions more Americans (around forty million, to be exact) could now be categorized as "clinically obese" due to the lowering of the standard BMI, thus qualifying them for those weight-loss drugs. Studies show that diet culture—which Harrison defines as "a system of beliefs that equates thinness, muscularity, and particular body shapes with health and moral virtue"—has had devastating consequences on people's mental, emotional, and physical health, and that weight-loss programs and restrictive dieting actually lead to weight *gain* for most people in the long run.

ANAD (the National Association for Anorexia Nervosa and Associated Disorders) reports that eating disorders affect 9 percent of the population worldwide and are the second-deadliest mental illness, secondary to opioid abuse. The eating disorder crisis disproportionately affects people with disabilities and LGBTQ+ folks, while BIPOC people are less likely to receive treatment. Meanwhile, diet culture is reaching even the youngest children; 42 percent of girls between first and third grade report wanting to be thinner.

So why is our culture so focused on losing weight when diet culture and the pressure to lose weight in many ways pose a greater risk to our health?

Because we live in a world shaped by Learned Hierarchical Beliefs—and in this paradigm, money, power, and status often override health, community, self-care, love, and safety. The "obesity epidemic" legend peddled by advertisers slinging the latest diet fads in magazines and on TV and social media, along with popular culture pushing out image after image of Eurocentric and fat-phobic body ideals, is imperative to maintaining the status quo of beauty hierarchy, moral hierarchy, the myth of laziness, unchecked individualism, and capitalism. Telling everyone that their mental and emotional health is far more important than how they look compared to an arbitrary standard rooted in racism, classism, and patriarchy doesn't maintain that status quo. An all-encompassing system structured around LHBs is dependent on you never feeling good enough.

I'm not saying that what we eat and how we care for our bodies shouldn't be part of the conversation. I'm saying that health is holistic, and what your body looks like is not an accurate measure of that health. Additionally, focusing on what you eat or how much you exercise as the only paths to health puts all the responsibility on the individual and ignores pervasive and toxic societal pressures that greatly influence our well-being, such as overwork, financial inequality, systemic racism and sexism, and lack of healthcare.

Using beauty standards as a means of establishing social, political, and economic hierarchies to control women's bodies and to devalue marginalized peoples as ugly, immoral, unintelligent, and a burden to society is an act of oppression. These toxic, unrealistic ideals have caused generations of people to suffer from poor self-image from the earliest ages. It saddens me to think about how so many of us, even as young children, looked in the mirror and hated what they saw.

I'd have done anything to get rid of my mustache.

"Oh my God, it turned black!" my little sister, Maria, screamed. I ran into the bathroom and saw a look of horror on her face. There was a grayish-black dark stain above her lip where she had just washed off the bleach cream we had bought at Sally's Beauty Supply earlier that day. Although the cream had bleached her upper lip hairs, it had had the reverse effect on her skin, creating an even stronger impression of a mustache than there had been before.

"What am I going to do now?" Maria asked the mirror, tears running down her face. The question seemed to not be directed at me or her reflection but at God himself. I knew her anguish all too well, and her terror that the dark stain above her lip would still be there by the time we went back to school on Monday.

My first attempt at conquering the battle against my body hair was plucking my mustache when I was ten, after a boy in my class had told me I needed to wax my upper lip. I sat on the bathroom counter with my feet in the sink to get really close to the mirror, and with my mother's tweezers extracted each little hair one by one.

Having unwanted body hair was something both of my sisters and I bonded over. When my older sister, Felili, started growing hair under her arms and thick hair on her legs when she hit puberty, my mom refused to let her shave it. Felili begged, she cried. But my mom didn't budge. She acted like shaving would open the door to premarital sex and a heroin addiction.

My mom didn't understand what it was like for us at school. Having hair on your body was one thing, but our body hair was dark and thick. When I saw the blond peach fuzz on my friends' legs, it looked like shimmers of gold in the sunlight; my hairs looked like someone had drawn little lines all over my legs with a Bic pen.

Body hair made me feel inferior, like there was something dirty or perverse about me. Like I wasn't feminine enough or there was something animalistic about me. I wanted to be accepted and to feel like I belonged. I wanted to look like the other girls.

Sometimes I imagine myself going back in time, visiting my younger self and saying, "I know you can't see it now, but you are so beautiful. And the ways you are different from those other girls are the most gorgeous things about you because they make you *you*."

Reframing Beauty

The first step to seeing beauty from the Higher Self perspective is to separate beauty standards (our culture's LHBs about physical appearance) from beauty. Beauty standards are barriers to seeing true beauty in yourself and in other people. They are like tunnel vision that blocks the entire spectrum of beauty from your awareness. For example, if you have been conditioned to believe that cellulite is unattractive, the moment you see cellulite on your body, your first thought might be *Eww.* When our consciousness is entrapped by LHBs, we see a reality that reflects those imposed beliefs. When we bring awareness to those LHBs, however, our perception begins to change. Rather than beauty being measured by where we score on a predetermined checklist (a checklist with a history of sexist, ableist, fatphobic, and racist oppression), we can create an opening to *recognizing* our Higher Selves—that is, seeing from a higher state of consciousness. *My LHBs say my cellulite is gross, but what would my Higher Self say? Perhaps that all my skin (including its texture and color) is a physical embodiment of my unique lineage, my humanness, an integral part of this sacred vessel that holds my spirit? That there is nothing gross about me?*

Recognizing beauty in ourselves isn't about being able to check off a list of beauty markers; it's seeing the natural radiance that exudes from our Higher Selves.

Now you might say, wait, there are evolutionary reasons why we are attracted to certain physical traits, which are based on our instincts to procreate and nurture and so on. To which I would argue that there is an evolutionary reason why we need to expand our awareness of the full spectrum of beauty: It is imperative for us to see the radiance in ourselves and each other and acknowledge that each one of us is an equally beautiful expression of the diversity of nature and the love of our Higher Selves, because our survival as a species depends on our ability to raise our consciousness to that of our Higher Selves. Otherwise, we will continue to create a world where we don't value ourselves and each other and therefore carry on our trajectory of unnecessary human suffering and the destruction of our planet and its vital resources.

When you see true beauty, you are seeing a person's spirit radiate from within.

Think about it: The more you love someone, the more beautiful they become in your eyes. That's because that love induces a state of your consciousness that actually expands your vision, enabling you to see the full spectrum of their beauty.

Our Learned Hierarchical Beliefs have given us tunnel vision, limiting our experience of beauty in this world. Despite this, beauty is all around us. When we are in the consciousness of love, we recognize beauty in each other. And in ourselves. When we lack the awareness of love, we don't actually experience beauty; we recognize beauty hierarchies and judge ourselves and each other accordingly.

Beauty isn't in the eye of the beholder—it's in the state of your consciousness.

These days, toxic beauty standards often lie hidden in wellness culture. When I lost a lot of weight doing yoga, I thought I was finally a healthy person. Because yoga is good for you. So the more yoga I did, the healthier I was, right?

Here's the deal: The choices you make for your body and health reflect the consciousness with which you make each choice. Higher-Selfing your body image means acknowledging that your choices need to come from a place of "I am already good enough," not "I need to do this to be good enough."

Making that distinction takes practice. And there is no shame if you are still unsure what those choices look like. It takes building awareness of the LHBs you carry with you that are putting a filter on your self-worth.

Beauty companies are expected to have spent $7.7 billion on advertising in 2022. That is a lot of money that is dependent on people wanting to change how they look. So, if you feel bad right now for judging your physical appearance, remember how deeply ingrained this stuff is in our collective history and the cultural messaging we consume every day.

It's important to remember that our LHBs about beauty are very powerful, and we shouldn't put an expectation on ourselves that just because we are aware of them we won't struggle with feeling inadequate when we look in the mirror. Shaming ourselves for not being able to see what we want to see in ourselves all the time is just another LHB trying to make us feel lacking. What our Higher Selves want us to do is be aware that those fears of not being good enough are not representative of the truth of who we are. They have been ingrained in us not just by the beauty industry, but also by the health and wellness industries. The more aware we are, the easier it is to have compassion for ourselves—and for others.

Aging

Our bodies change; they are always in a process of transformation. Our culture, because it has become so fixated on looking young, suffers from ageism. People are terrified of their changing, aging bodies. The beauty industry profits off those fears by pushing products with so-called anti-aging formulas.

Our bodies are not supposed to stay the same over the years. We aren't supposed to always be the same weight. The texture of our skin may change, and some of us lose hair or grow hair in places we never had it before. Some of us get varicose veins, or additional freckles and spots. Watching our bodies change isn't a sign that something is wrong. Because our culture treats aging as if it's a bad thing, there isn't enough discussion about the natural physical changes we can expect as we age. So many of us are caught off-guard. The more we talk about them, the easier it will be to honor them.

Imagine if popular culture truly embraced the beauty of aging instead of constantly trying to sell us products that tried to prevent it! Remember, seeing the full spectrum of beauty is a shift in your consciousness. When you look in the mirror and see wrinkles on your face and immediately judge them as bad—what consciousness are you in? **Who put that message in your head?**

It's Okay to Want to Change

What we see is a result of our state of consciousness. Does that mean that if we want to change or alter our bodies, we don't love ourselves? No, it doesn't. It just means that however your body looks, whatever shape it takes, is beautiful because of who you are. If altering your body helps you to feel more aligned with your Higher Self, then that is your choice alone. You know what is best for you.

Many trans and nonbinary folks who experience gender dysphoria feel much more themselves after undergoing physical transformation. These changes in appearance help them channel their Higher Selves by aligning how they feel inside with how they see themselves on the outside. The desire to change how you look becomes harmful only when you judge those characteristics based on a hierarchy. You were beautiful before you changed, and you are beautiful now.

When we channel who we really are, we radiate. When we see someone for who they really are, we see the magnificent creature they were created to be.

The first time I felt truly beautiful was when I realized that every part of me from my nose to my toes deserved to be here. That my body was unlike any other body in this world. Isn't it amazing that there are so many of us and yet we all look exactly like ourselves?

Understanding that we are so much more than our bodies actually helps us honor them and treat them with love, compassion, patience, and gratitude. Our bodies are gifts.

Nowadays, I have to be really mindful when I get into a workout routine, and make sure to check in on what is motivating me. Having a healthy body has shifted for me from the goal of looking a certain way to seeing myself through the lens of my Higher Self. From that perspective, I can make choices about my body that come from love, not a desire to fulfill someone else's definition of worth or a bout of self-loathing during which I deny my body the nourishment it needs.

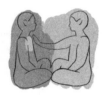

Your Higher Self in Body Image and Beauty Standards

1. **When you criticize how you look in a mirror, ask yourself,** *Where is this thought coming from?* We've all done it: Seen a glimpse of ourselves in the mirror or a photo we are in and cringed. First, I just want to acknowledge literally how mean that is. Imagine someone walking by you and cringing out loud at how you look. Just. Mean. You would probably never do that to another person, yet you would do that to yourself. You deserve better! Secondly, it's understandable to criticize how you look, because you've been conditioned to do so. You can practice becoming aware of these critical thoughts and asking yourself where they came from. My LHBs about body hair? My conditioned fatphobia? The voice of some kid at school who told me I was ugly? It's not about making those thoughts wrong or bad. It's about noticing them and getting curious as to why they're there. Soon you will see you have more choice in the thoughts you choose to believe than you realized.

2. **How you see yourself depends on your state of consciousness.** Have you ever looked at old pictures of yourself and thought, *Wow, I looked good!* only to remember how bad you felt when they were taken? Has a friend or loved one ever criticized their body in front of you, while you thought, *You look amazing!* Valuing ourselves isn't about changing how we look on the outside; it's about changing our perspective inside. That is the key to a peaceful and holistic relationship with how you see your physical body. It's not about always "loving" the way you look; it's about acknowledging that your conditioning affects how you perceive yourself. And that your Higher Self is the part of you that *knows* that you are beautiful just how you are. That is your truth.

3. **What you see in other people also depends on your state of consciousness.** Who hasn't compared how they look to someone else and felt inadequate? That is a result of you seeing that person through the lens of your LHBs — how close or far away they are from the standard of beauty you have been conditioned to believe in. Sometimes you perceive them as closer to that standard than yourself and sometimes farther away. In other words, someone is either better looking or not. From the Higher Self perspective, recognizing beauty in another person is not seeing them as better or worse. It's seeing them in their unique radiance, an outer expression of their inner value. Their beauty does not negate your own. When I am really channeled into my Higher Self, it's amazing how much beauty I see in the people around me.

4. **Educate yourself on diet culture.** Diet culture impacts our lives in ways we don't often notice because it's a part of the world we were born into. But you can educate yourself on the facts. Does not eating gluten really make you healthy? Is the latest diet fad just another way the industry is trying to profit from your insecurities? I'd recommend learning about

diet culture from experts and doctors who specialize in disordered eating. Facts about the harm that diets cause is not the messaging that normally appears in your Instagram algorithm. We must seek it out. In the Notes section of this chapter I have included some accounts I have found helpful when addressing diet culture.

5. **Don't make assumptions about other people's bodies.** Again, weight is not an accurate measure of health, despite what we have been trained to think.

6. **Nourishment doesn't just come from "healthy" food.** Self-compassion, kindness, acceptance, and love are vital nourishment for your health. It's wonderful to eat all the nutrients that keep your body healthy, but you counter that effort when you emotionally abuse your body at the same time.

7. **If you are struggling with disordered eating, you deserve help, support, and guidance.** You are not alone. Many people struggle privately, worried about being judged for their struggles with food. They spend years suffering alone. I'm here to tell you that you are beautiful. That everyone's wounds manifest differently, and just because yours do in this area of your life does not mean there is something wrong with you, that you are weak or immoral. Please reach out for help. In the Notes section of this chapter, I have included some resources.

Reminders

- Stop using other people as a mirror to project the delusion that you are inadequate.
- The next time you feel insecure, remember our culture manufactures insecurity and you have been consuming an illusion — the illusion that you are not inherently worthy and beautiful.
- Love expands your vision to see the full spectrum of beauty. Beauty standards are culturally enforced tunnel vision.

- Our culture conditions us to feel unworthy, then tells us there is something wrong with us for struggling with self-worth. Stop judging yourself for having a hard time. You are not the problem.

Affirmations

- All my features make me beautiful because they make me *me*.
- Beauty standards could never encapsulate my beauty.
- My insecurities are not telling me the truth.
- I don't have to believe every thought I have.
- This body is a sacred vessel for my divine spirit.
- I see so much beauty all around me.

Writing Exercise

Write a love letter to your body. Tell it all the things you are grateful for about it. For example, you could say, "Thank you for letting me taste yummy food." Or, "Thank you for working so hard to heal my cold." Tell it you are sorry for being so critical and insulting. Our bodies are constantly working on our behalf, but we rarely honor them. When you are done, put the letter in a special place. You can always add to it or take it out if you are ever in a place where you notice you have been really hard on your body.

Journal Prompts

1. LHBs that I carry with me about my beauty and body image are...

2. Those thoughts were put into my head by...

3. Flip the script: My Higher Self would respond to those
    thoughts by saying...

    _____

4. I feel most beautiful when...

    _____

5. My definition of beauty is...

    _____

6. I am beautiful because...

    _____

Chapter 13

Sex and Pleasure

Me: *Why is it embarrassing to talk about my own sexual pleasure?*

Higher Self: *Because the patriarchy has conditioned you to believe it is shameful, when it's really an act of self-care.*

I've done a very bad thing.

Staring into the stained-glass portrait of Jesus one Sunday at church when I was in the fourth grade, I contemplated the very bad thing I had done the previous day: looking up s-e-x in the dictionary in my bedroom while my family was downstairs watching the football game. When I first looked up s-e-x, it just said something about being male or female. But then it said "see—sexual intercourse." So I went further down the page and looked up sexual intercourse, and it said the penis goes inside the vagina. *The guy's part goes inside the girl's part?* My Barbies had had s-e-x since preschool, since my cousin showed me how to rub Ken and Barbie up and down together. So that's what I thought it was. After I read this new information in the dictionary, I started to feel weird *down there*. So I put my stuffed animal between my legs.

A couple of months prior, at my friend Emily's house, we had played truth or dare. When it was my turn, Emily dared me to hump the couch in her den. I had no idea what she meant, so she showed me. That's what I had done the day before; I humped my big stuffed animal, and felt a rush like electricity was traveling through my body all the way to my fingertips. It felt so good, but afterward I felt so bad. I felt wrong. Thankfully no one in my family had caught me, but what if God was watching? He probably thought I was a big pervert. I imagined the pastor below us stopping the sermon and pointing up to me in the audience and saying, "Jesus saw what you did!" But instead, he just told the congregation to stand and sing a

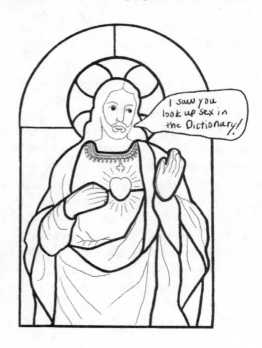

hymn. "Praise God from whom all blessings flow. Praise Him all creatures here below..." As I sang, I made a promise to Jesus that I'd never hump again.

We Were Not Taught About Pleasure

LHBs rooted in religious oppression, patriarchy, racism, homophobia, and transphobia have shaped our cultural narrative on sexual pleasure and desire. Centuries of religious dogma taught us that sex was for the purpose of procreation, not pleasure. Racism and colorism perpetuated myths of the supposed animalistic and uncivilized sexual desire of BIPOCs while exoticizing and sexually exploiting Black and Brown bodies. At various times participating in sexual activity between two consenting adults outside of the cis heteronormative framework—that is, for the purposes of pleasure only—was illegal. Doctors and scientists' patriarchal assumptions on sexuality maintained a narrative that sexual desire was not as pronounced in female-assigned bodies as it was in males. Homosexual desire was labeled pathological. We carry with us literally hundreds of years of religious, psychological, and pseudoscientific hierarchical conditioning and misinformation about sexual pleasure.

We were also raised by caregivers who passed down to us their LHBs about sex and pleasure. Many of us grew up in strict traditional homes that condemned and punished any sexual activity before marriage. Parental figures rarely, if ever, engaged us in discussions about masturbation, despite those experiences being a completely natural curiosity and part of our sexual development. The less we heard about sex, the more we interpreted it as something that was not to be talked about, something that was inappropriate, which is to say, wrong. The more we were made to feel that our sexuality was something to be ashamed of, the less safe we felt asking for guidance and support.

Sadly, many of us also grew up with experiences of sexual trauma. Often we felt responsible for our own trauma due to victim-shaming, manipulation, gaslighting, and narratives promoting the viewpoint that sexual assault accusations would unfairly ruin the perpetrators' lives. We took on feelings of unworthiness along with psychological, physical, and emotional wounds. We learned to dissociate from our bodies for our own survival.

In school many of us were taught about abstinence and about the dangers and risks of sex, but never about pleasure, love, and what consensual and safe experiences looked like. We were never told that sexual pleasure was a good thing. Which made it even harder to navigate what to do with our feelings and curiosities and how to honor the changes in our bodies without shaming ourselves.

Despite very little open and honest discussion about sex and pleasure, gender biases about sex seeped into our psyches at a young age. We watched movies and TV that depicted women as sexual objects and men who earned their merit based on sexual conquests. The all-too-common double standard that women taking pleasure in sexual behavior were sluts and men taking pleasure should be celebrated played out in social dynamics in school as soon as we reached puberty.

STD (sluts toking dope)

"For a good time call 214-555-5555."

I arrived at my eighth grade social studies class one day and found a note in my desk with this message. It was meant for me to find, because it was my phone number on the note. I had no idea who wrote it. But I'd gotten used to things like that. Since the second semester of sixth grade, I had been labeled a slut. When I first heard the term I was surprised, because at the time I had only kissed a boy once. It had happened at a party during a game called Seven Minutes in Heaven. His name was Benji.

I had had a crush on him since the second grade. I don't even think our mouths opened when we kissed. And a month after that I had a different boyfriend. So I guess the combination of the kiss and the new boyfriend made people think I was a slut?

Eventually I made friends with a group of girls who were also known as sluts at our school: Crystal, Meg, and Abby. We were like a little crew. People thought Crystal was a slut because she was dating a ninth-grader. Meg got called a slut because there was a rumor she gave two different guys a blowjob at a party. (I don't know if it was true—I've never asked.) And Abby...well, I'm not sure why Abby was considered a slut. Maybe because she had a single mom who drank and her older sister had something of a reputation, or maybe it was just that she was friends with us. Crystal, Meg, and Abby and I started calling ourselves STD. It stood for "sluts toking dope." It was our way of defending ourselves from the social shaming—to act like we were proud of it. So I started doing a lot of sexual stuff with boys. I made out, got felt up, was fingered (God, I hate that word, but that was what people called it), and jerked off a boy at a movie theater. I had to go to the bathroom and get us a bunch of paper towels to clean up.

Growing up socialized as a girl, you are made to feel like you're a slut if you do sexual stuff with boys, but you also feel like it's what you are supposed to do. I had no concept of sexual activity for enjoyment. If I had been told, "Hey, sex is supposed to feel good," I might have asked myself the question, *Why am I doing this if it's not pleasurable?*

Accessing Pleasure and Eroticism

With all the LHBs we grew up with about sexual desire, and a culture that puts productivity ahead of joy and self-care, is it any wonder many of us feel a lack of connection to what is pleasurable to us? Is it any surprise that many of us don't communicate with our sexual partners about what we want in bed, or find it difficult to explore our own sexual curiosities? When we have been taught to associate erotic desire with feelings of guilt, unworthiness, or even danger, it's no wonder we feel guilty and unworthy of pleasure, and also distrust our own bodies and feelings. Not only do we feel fearful of discovering what feels good, but we convince ourselves we don't deserve to feel good.

Sexual experiences can also bring LHBs about body image and self-worth to the surface. *I'm not sexy enough. I don't look good naked. I'm not good enough for this person. I'm not lovable.* It's easy to get consumed in these thoughts. Physical intimacy can be an extremely vulnerable experience, and without the empowerment of your Higher Self, we can get so caught up in our LHBs that joy and pleasure seem out of reach. Connecting to your Higher Self is acknowledging that those LHBs are not telling you the truth. From the Higher Self perspective, pleasure is an experience of your wholeness, the recognition that all the parts of you are valuable, sacred, and deserving of joy. Exploring your erotic nature—including your imagination, your fantasies, your desires, and what feels good in your body—is a practice in self-acceptance, because you are actively rejecting the LHBs that told you you shouldn't feel good about your sexuality, that you should feel guilty for wanting pleasure, and that your sexual desires are shameful. **Pleasure isn't something you need to prove you are worthy of, because it is part of who you are. It is feeling the joy of your aliveness and receiving the gifts your body and spirit have to offer you.**

In Audre Lorde's essay "Uses of the Erotic: The Erotic as Power," she describes eroticism as a spiritual resource within ourselves that must be reclaimed from oppressive forces that have attempted to suppress it. The erotic, according to Lorde, encompasses much more than sexual desire—it is a "provocative force" beyond sensation to the "depths of feeling." The erotic can be made manifest in all our endeavors when we channel the fullest expression of our wholeness and intuitive wisdom — in other words, when we desire ourselves.

Likewise, our Higher Selves encompass the parts of us that are aware of our inner worth. Exploring our sexuality and erotic desires is a sacred expression of our awakening. Allowing pleasure and joy in our lives is affirming that we have always deserved it.

If you are in a time in your life where accessing pleasure and feeling empowered about your sexuality is challenging, it doesn't mean anything is wrong with you! That is just another sneaky LHB trying to make you feel less-than. The first step to channeling your erotic power is to fully accept that wherever you are in your sexual journey is okay. And no matter what LHBs you are working on letting go of as a result of our culture or the trauma you have been through, it doesn't mean those LHBs define your sexuality. Your erotic power comes from within — it is part of who you are, and there is nothing that anyone can do or say to change that.

When you give yourself grace and compassion, taking steps to experience more pleasure becomes less challenging. Your Higher Self is essential to channeling your erotic power, because the LHBs that disempower us sexually need to be brought to light. That doesn't mean insecurities will never come up. It means that when they do you will begin asking yourself, *Who is talking here? Is it my internalized shame, or my Higher Self that knows, no matter what, I am whole and worthy of joy?* Whenever you accept yourself — all of yourself, including your wounds and the things you are working on letting go of — you have stepped into your power, because you are acknowledging that even though there are things you are working on unlearning, you are willing to unlearn them *because* you deserve pleasure without shame! You're already doing it!

The Joy of Self-Discovery

Pleasure looks and feels different to different people because we come from different experiences, we have different relationships to our bodies, and we are in different stages of unlearning and healing. What is pleasurable to you might not be to someone else. And that is okay! That is why self-pleasure is so helpful when it comes to understanding what feels right in your body. We grew up with such a lack of information and also disinformation when it came to sexual anatomy and function. It's not uncommon for people, especially those socialized as female, to either be complacent with a level of ignorance about their bodies/sexuality or have feelings of fear or disgust about their own anatomy and sexual function. Shame is so insidious, it will have us believing that the way we were created was fundamentally wrong or bad. The sex educator and author Emily Nagoski, in her book *Come As You Are*, recommends a practice to help nurture your relationship to your most intimate parts: taking a hand mirror or the camera on your phone and propping it up to look at your genitals. If the idea of doing that makes you feel uneasy, ask yourself, *Who or what taught me to fear my own body?*

Thankfully there are a lot more resources available to educate yourself about your body, about other people's bodies, and about different ways to experience pleasure, including books, websites dedicated to sexual education, and how-to videos, toys to experiment with, and sex educators to follow on social media. It's never too late to expand your understanding of yourself and explore how your sexuality could be more joyfully expressed. Self-pleasure is self-care!

Talking About Pleasure

Many of us have been in situations where we were engaged in sexual activity with a partner or partners and we wanted to be more vocal about what was working for us and what wasn't. And I'm sure a lot of us have also been engaged in sexual activity where we wanted our partner to give us more direction when it came to pleasing them. But often we feel too shy to speak out or too insecure to ask someone what they want because we feel like we are just supposed to know somehow. Look, no one taught us how to talk about sex or even how to have pleasurable sex, so if both of those are a struggle for you, it makes a lot of sense!

We need to approach these conversations from the lens of our Higher Selves. Everyone carries with them their own set of LHBs and fears of inadequacy. We need to speak with care and tenderness. We need to do our best to be a safe space for someone to be open and honest about their feelings and boundaries and never shame anyone's fantasies, desires, or kinks. There is a difference between saying you are not interested in something and making someone feel like there is something wrong with them. Simply being honest about the challenges of talking about sex is an opening to deeper communication. Let's say for example that there is something you have wanted from a partner sexually but don't know how to ask for it. Rather than going straight for what you want to ask for, it can often be helpful to have a discussion *about* discussing sex with your partner. Something like, "I've been wanting to be more open about what my desires and fantasies are when it comes to our sex, but it's not always easy for me to bring it up because, you know, our culture puts so much shame on us sexually and no one taught us how to talk about this stuff. I'd love to hear about what you really like in bed and also to tell you what I really like." The bonus about being vulnerable and honest is it helps other people open up and feel more comfortable in their honesty and vulnerability with you. If you're not interested in that approach, start with vocalizing what you do like, for example, "I really like it when you touch me this way . . . " or "This feels really good." It can also help to talk with positive affirmation when asking your sexual partners questions — for example, "Does that feel good?" When you are mustering up the courage to talk about what you want, keep in mind that you deserve pleasure just like anyone else. And if something you want is new or different from what a partner wants, that is okay! Most of all, remember that people want to feel accepted for who they are — and it's from that place you can start communicating more openly and collaborating on joyful and fun sexual experiences.

Sexual Boundaries

Your Higher Self knows you are deserving of care, respect, and safety when it comes to your sexual experiences with other partners, and that means thinking deeply about what boundaries will help you stay in your power. "Sex positivity" is a term that is often used to negate the puritanical shame our culture puts on us when it comes to exploring our sexuality. Sometimes people misinterpret sex positivity to mean that you are so positive about sex that you have minimal boundaries. But boundaries help us to have more positive sexual experiences because they create a secure foundation for you to be in touch with your erotic power. You can think of them as your own personal guidelines on your sexual journey. For example, one boundary could be that you don't hook up with someone on the first day you meet them, not because there is something morally wrong with it but because in past experiences it hasn't worked well for you, or you need to know more about the person to see if you're compatible and one date isn't enough. Another boundary could be a sex act that you do not want to do when you are hooking up. "I'm not into that" is a clear way to communicate that boundary. Maybe at first you thought you were interested in doing something in bed but then discovered you're not.

It's never too late to communicate a boundary! It's never too late to say no. Likewise, understanding a sexual partner's boundaries and honoring them is vital to consent. RAINN, the United States' largest anti–sexual violence organization, defines consent as "an affirmative agreement between participants to engage in physical or sexual activity." They emphasize that consent is a constant conversation, with both parties asking each other what they are comfortable with before moving forward. For example, asking, "Is it okay if I kiss you?" or "Can I touch you there?"

Vocalizing your boundaries and asking about a partner's boundaries might not feel easy at first. But the more you remind yourself that your needs are important and that boundaries empower you to have more joyful sexual experiences, the easier it gets. Your boundaries are up to you to decide, and they can evolve as you grow to know more about what makes you feel comfortable. But what is most important is that consent is established and your boundaries are respected and honored by the people you choose to share space with.

Spirituality Is Not Separate from Sexuality

Organized religion has attempted to separate sexual expression from the realm of the sacred, so it's not a surprise that we often think that sexual pleasure has no connection to our spiritual path. However, since ancient times, merging the sexual with the sacred has been practiced in spiritual traditions and rituals, particularly in Eastern religions such as Hinduism and Buddhism. Some practitioners of Western occultism beginning in the nineteenth century used a sexual ritual called sex magik as an opening to higher states of consciousness and manifestation.

From the Higher Self perspective, sexuality is an important facet of spirituality because pleasure can be used as a transcendent experience for moving beyond total identification with the body. Using your physical body as a portal to feeling the aliveness of your inner being can bring you to a state of presence with your Higher Self, similar to meditation. From that place you are disidentified with your LHBs, you are merging with the consciousness of love and the awareness of your wholeness. Using sexual expression as a spiritual practice is a tradition that has been practiced for centuries, and finding new ways to implement that in your life can be a beautiful way to honor your sacred eroticism.

Honor Yourself

Our Higher Selves can help us stay grounded in our worth no matter where we are in our sexual journeys. The point isn't for everything to always be functioning perfectly. The point is that approaching sex and pleasure with the consciousness of self-acceptance gives you permission to keep healing. You deserve safe, loving, and joyful sexual experiences, whether that is with another person, with multiple people, or with yourself. **Pleasure is amazing. Pleasure is revolutionary. Pleasure is healing.** But just because it is sometimes difficult to access does not make you any less powerful or valuable. You were created whole. You are a gift. And you are always deserving of joy.

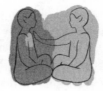

Bring Your Higher Self to Sex and Pleasure

1. **Healthy sexuality does not look the same for everyone.** Who you have sex with, how often, in what position, whether you are monogamous or polyamorous, whether you are into sex parties, kink, or only solo play, whether you partake in one-night stands or date someone for a long time before having sex — it's all about what feels right for you. There is no one path to aligning with your erotic power. Even a one-night stand can be a sacred experience. What matters is where your heart is. The more connected you stay with your Higher Self, the more you nurture your self-acceptance and awareness of your wholeness — and the more you will trust yourself and make choices about your sexuality that reflect your self-worth. Sex positivity comes from the inside out. Not the outside in.

2. **Sexual trauma does not define your sexuality.** There is nothing easy about healing from sexual trauma. It's one of the darkest aspects of our unhealed world, affecting a huge

proportion of our global population. But no matter what anyone has ever done to you or any experience you have had, you are whole, pure, divine, and lovable. You deserve support in your healing. And you have every right to experience joy and pleasure as much as anyone else. Our wounds are not who we are.

3. **Fantasies are cool.** I am a highly visual person. I have a vivid imagination. I used to feel ashamed of having sexual fantasies. Traditional Christian doctrine often condemned even the thoughts of sexual experiences, not just the acts. People go to priests to confess their "impure" thoughts. This has had devastating psychological and spiritual effects on many people. Fantasies do not make you bad; they do not make you wrong. You are allowed to have an internal erotic life that you share with others or keep completely to yourself. You should never condemn yourself for having fantasies.

4. **Talking about what you want in bed can feel hard, but it's also important and gets easier with practice.** For some people, telling their partners what they like and don't like can feel paralyzing. But there is nothing shameful or wrong about sexual desire. It's really important to facilitate a safe space for ourselves and our partners to talk about sex. To never shame another person about what they like even if you aren't into it, or let other people shame you. Sex and pleasure are very sensitive subjects for many people, so being mindful, caring, and compassionate with ourselves and others is key.

Affirmations

- There is nothing shameful about my pleasure.
- Every time I give myself love I am embodied in my erotic power.
- My sexuality is sacred.
- Nothing that anyone said or did could take away from my self-worth.

- I deserve to have my boundaries honored and respected no matter what.
- I am on a journey of self-discovery. I trust myself.
- I can enjoy the moment.
- I am allowed to indulge.

Journal Prompts

1. My fears or insecurities around sex and pleasure are...

   _____

2. Some experiences or beliefs that could be contributing to those fears are...

   _____

3. Things I could tell myself to lessen that fear are...

   _____

4. Some sexual experiences I would like to have in the future are...

   _____

5. My sexual needs and boundaries are valid because...

   _____

Chapter 14

Queerness and the Gender Spectrum

> **Me:** *Someone told me that I'm too feminine to be nonbinary.*
>
> **Higher Self:** *Nonbinary means you don't identify with the social construct of the binary, the same construct that says men have to look one way and women have to look the other. How you identify is not based on how you look, but how you feel inside. No one knows who you are better than you.*

What are little boys made of?
Frogs and snails and puppy-dogs' tails.
That's what little boys are made of.
What are little girls made of?
Sugar and spice and all things nice.
That's what little girls are made of.
—Nineteenth-century nursery rhyme

Gender in Service to LHBs

Gender roles—the behaviors and characteristics that are socially constructed to differentiate people who are assigned male and female at birth—are not at face-value harmful. They become harmful when used in service of patriarchal, racist, homophobic, and transphobic LHBs, which has been the case for countless generations. We have been taught to believe the gender assigned to us by society is who we are. Rather than seeing gender expression as an individual choice, we are told to define ourselves according to social constructs dictated by LHBs; therefore our authenticity, self-expression, and freedoms have been stifled, including the freedom to wear what we want to wear, pursue the interests and passions we want to pursue, earn as much money as we deserve, and love who we want to love.

According to a hierarchical belief system, the more you fit into culturally accepted gender roles, the better you are—the more whole you are. And people that don't fit in are therefore less worthy. At various times in human history, people who defied the rules of gender—for example, wives refusing to submit to their husbands, men wearing skirts in public, and individuals partaking in homosexual relationships—were labeled immoral, mentally unstable, criminal, sexually deviant, and a danger to society. Punishments included social ridicule, imprisonment, torture, and even death. For Black people and people of color, defying rules of gender poses higher risk, because racism adds another layer to the perceived "threat" that self-empowerment through self-determination poses to a hierarchical system.

Gender Is a Spectrum

From the Higher Self perspective, gender is a spectrum of self-expression. There is no right or wrong way to perform gender. How we choose to present ourselves in the world has no bearing on our self-worth or our value. We were born whole and deserving of love. Gender expression is a medium for feeling more connected to our authenticity—in other words, our Higher Selves, or who we are beyond the limitations of a hierarchical and oppressive belief system. What clothes you wear, what your interests are, and how you see yourself in relation to the community around you is a reflection of your inner world. When gender roles dictated by society put limits on our outer expression, it is an attempt to hinder self-discovery, because the more we are in touch with our truth, with our Higher Selves, the more we will question the LHBs that have kept oppressive forces in power.

Queer and trans people are at the forefront of expanding our awareness of who we are beyond society's gender "norms." And because of that they are feared, scapegoated, and misunderstood by those who want to maintain the status quo.

Finding my truth

I never officially came out. When I was fifteen my mom caught me kissing my girlfriend in my high school parking lot. I had forgotten she was picking me up from school for a doctor's appointment. She pulled up right when Kim and I had our tongues down each other's throat, leaning on Kim's 'eighty-nine Volvo.

Both of my parents refused to accept my queer relationship, claiming that I wasn't actually gay and that they didn't allow gay people in their house. But I kept seeing my girlfriend. For months, I was fighting with them. I'd run away from home and stay at my girlfriend's house, then return and end up getting kicked out again.

Eventually, my mom tried a different tack: She took me to a therapist.

When we pulled up to the office for my first appointment, I was shocked to see that it wasn't a professional building. It was a house.

"Why is it at a house?" I asked.

"He was highly recommended," my mom said. "I'll pick you up in forty-five minutes."

A white-haired old man who looked like Colonel Sanders opened the front door to greet me.

"Hello, I'm Dr. Harris, it's nice to meet you. Come on in."

I walked into a dark house with forest green walls, maroon curtains, and lots of antique-looking furniture. It reminded me of the period films my mom and I loved to watch, and for a moment I imagined I was being led into some nineteenth-century all-girls boarding school where I would learn Latin, drink tea, and play croquet.

He led me into the dining room and told me to take a seat at a large mahogany table. At the end of the table was an easel with one of those jumbo pads of paper on it. He sat in a chair next to the easel and proceeded to ask me a lot of questions about how I grew up, my relationship with my parents, particularly my dad, and different struggles my family had had.

"Did you get much attention from your father growing up?" "How often were your parents at home?" "How well do you get along with your mom?"

After I tried to answer his questions the best I could, he stood up and started drawing a sort of map on the pad of paper, kind of like a family tree, listing out my family members and different events I had told him about during our talk.

He explained to me that I wasn't actually gay, but that my relationship with my dad and the struggles I'd had with my parents over the years were making me think I was gay. Because what I really wanted was my dad's love and attention.

When my mom picked me up from the appointment, I felt humiliated.

"I'm never going back there," I told her.

I could see the disappointment in her eyes. Like she expected me to get into the car and say, "Mom, you were right. I'm not gay after all."

As we drove away in silence, I couldn't help feeling sorry for her. I was supposed to marry a man and have kids. I was supposed to make her proud. What would she tell her side of the family? What would people think? Intuitively I knew that her fears had much more to do with her than me.

Belonging

Our Learned Hierarchical Beliefs have created a world in which some people are told they don't belong: to womanhood, to manhood, to girlhood, to boyhood, to society, to their families, to what is normal, what is valid, what is moral, what is real. Queer and trans people are told to deny their deepest feelings and intuition, to ignore what their hearts are telling them in order to be accepted. This has less to do with who they are attracted to or how they identify than it does with the threat that they pose to a hierarchical belief system that is dependent on the suppression of our Higher Selves in order to sustain itself.

Queer, trans, and gender-nonconforming people existing in their authenticity exposes not only gender bias, homophobia, and transphobia, but also the unconscious fears non-queer people have of living authentically. Everyone, no matter what society labels you as, suffers from a world where some people belong and some don't, where some people deserve to live and some don't, because the message it sends is "You can't be yourself here." We have been conditioned to hide parts of ourselves, to limit self-discovery and self-expression so that we can fit into the status quo and be accepted; otherwise we will be perceived as a threat. It is no coincidence that when queer, trans, and gender-nonconforming people are openly embracing themselves and shining their light, they are most at risk of violence, as was the case with the tragic murder of O'Shae Sibley, a Black queer man who was fatally stabbed to death in Brooklyn after voguing to Beyoncé with his friends at a gas station. The idea that someone could be queer *and* love themselves threatens the hierarchical belief system that so many people cling to. Without being better than queer and trans people, without an "other" to look down on, they don't know what their worth is. They feel powerless. And so harming and harassing queer, trans, and gender-nonconforming people is a desperate attempt to feel powerful again.

But our Higher Selves are more powerful than LHBs. So powerful that in the face of rejection and social ridicule, even children and young people follow the guidance of their hearts. It is their Higher Selves that empower them to come out as queer and trans and to stand up in the face of opposition for their right to love who they want and to be who they are. When I think about coming out as a teen and the struggles I had with my parents, although it was a sad and traumatic experience I shouldn't have had to go through, I am also so proud of my ability to harness my Higher Self and get in touch with my truth, regardless of the conversion therapist who gaslighted me and the destabilization of losing the unconditional acceptance of my parents. I had the love and acceptance of my Higher Self, and that carried me through.

Beyond the Binary

Queer and trans people have always existed, long before the arrival of European settler colonists, long before the pathologizing of selfhood by Western medicine. People who possessed qualities outside of a binary understanding of male and female have been revered by many North American Native tribes for centuries. Known today under the umbrella term of Two Spirit, they were often put in positions of leadership because of their perceived spiritual insights. The origin of my indigenous heritage, Samoa, has traditionally recognized a third gender named *fa'afafine*. These are people who are assigned male at birth but who possess what are characterized as feminine affectations and behaviors. Other non-Western cultures around the world have recognized gender outside the binary of male and female for centuries, such as the *hijras* in Hindu society, the *muxes* of the indigenous Zapotec people in Mexico, and the *sekrata* of the Sakalava, indigenous to Madagascar. In a white supremacist and transphobic culture, it's no wonder this more expansive understanding of gender was not part of our Western education.

In addition to gender, we are also taught that sex can exist only as a binary. We were assigned male or female at birth based on our anatomy: XX chromosomes for female, XY for male, a uterus and ovaries for female, a penis and scrotum for male. However, 2 percent of the population are born with variations of that binary sex definition. Examples of this include a person born with the chromosomes of a female but genitalia that appear male, or an infant born with XY chromosomes and a uterus. "Intersex" is a comprehensive term for a variety of sex anatomy. There are "over 30 medical terms for specific characteristics of intersex traits," according to InterAct, an organization that advocates for intersex youth.

Since the 1950s, doctors have performed surgeries on infants and children to "normalize" their sex as either male or female, including reducing the size of the clitoris, leading to recorded instances of psychological and physical trauma. Many intersex activists are advocating to end these so-called corrective surgeries on infants and children until they are old enough to make the decision for themselves, especially since the majority of intersex conditions pose no medical risk. Despite intersex people being about as common statistically as redheads, the biological "fact" that there are only two sexes is still taught every day in schools.

For far too long our hierarchical culture has attempted to erase the existence of trans and gender-nonconforming people to enforce a binary gender system in an attempt to limit our self-actualization through oppressive laws, public shaming, gaslighting, medical intervention, punishment, and violence. The consequences have not only been devastating to queer, trans, and gender-nonconforming

people, but have perpetuated the illusion that in order to be lovable and worthy you need to hide yourself, make yourself smaller,
and hinder your spirit. As the gender-nonconforming activist and
poet Alok Van Menon so beautifully articulated, "When they
[transphobic and homophobic people] see us trans and gender
non-conforming people have the audacity to be free, to actually live
the lives that they thought and still think are impossible, lives that
are curated and cultivated around joy and possibility and expansion, they perceive us as a threat and not an invitation to another
way to be."

Our Higher Selves know that humanity could never be limited to a binary understanding of gender and sexuality because not
everyone fits into that mold. And all of us were created whole. All
of us are a gift to this world just for being who we are. Honoring
the spectrum of our unique identities is an act of love, not just for
your fellow humans but also for yourself, because you are affirming that everyone including you is worthy of acceptance, compassion, and respect. We are not separate.

Nonbinary spirit

For as long as I can remember, I've felt *different* when it
came to gender. Like the outside of me (how I presented myself
gender-wise) didn't encapsulate how I felt inside. Sometimes I
felt like a boy on the inside, even though I didn't want to look
like a boy in the typical binary way. The first time I heard the
term "nonbinary," something clicked inside me. I felt an opening within me that I hadn't felt before. *Could I be nonbinary?* I
was nervous that people even in the queer community would
judge me the same way as my parents had when I came out
as gay. I thought that because I was so feminine-presenting, I
couldn't be nonbinary. But connecting to my Higher Self—who
I am beyond conditioning, labels, even identities—helped me

realize that how I wanted to express my authenticity was with whatever labels helped me to feel free.

For me, nonbinary is a reflection of my spirit, and my spirit is beyond gender and sex, so nonbinary feels right for me.

We all have different reasons for identifying the way we do. We can honor our identities without disrespecting or belittling or denying others the right to honor theirs. If there is one thing I know for sure, it's that language is incredibly limiting. One word could never encompass the wholeness of who we all are. Neither could our anatomy, or our chromosomes.

If history teaches us anything, it's that our understanding of the concepts of sex and gender is always expanding and evolving. And so is how we see ourselves and each other.

We Are All Gifts

Our Higher Selves know that every life is sacred and that everyone belongs. We can create a world where everyone has the freedom to fully express the truth of their hearts, a world where we believe people when they tell us who they are, a world where we protect each other from harm, a world where people come out from the shadows of their LHBs and step into the empowerment of their Higher Selves. It starts with each of us being willing to let love be our guide.

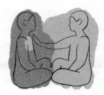

Bring Your Higher Self to Your Relationship to Queerness and Gender

1. **Remember that even though we live in a homophobic, transphobic, patriarchal system, most people love and accept people for who they are.** Hatred is so loud these days. It seems like everywhere in the media there is some jerk making a sexist remark. Or an internet troll saying something awful on the post of a trans person just trying to live their life. Have you ever looked at the comment section of a post and found that despite hundreds of loving and encouraging comments from people, the few sexist or anti-queer comments are the ones that pull your focus? Our animal brains are trained to look out for danger. So it makes sense that what we see as a threat stands out way more than the countless acts of love that are far more common — I mean far, far more common. Part of our Higher Self work is to actively remember that. To notice love more. It's our evolutionary step out of the animal brain. To see it in the places you might normally overlook. I promise you it's there. People want you to succeed. They want you to be happy and healthy. Because they want that for themselves too. There are so many beautiful humans in our world who are growing and unlearning with you. Don't forget that.

2. **Queerness and gender identity are about how you feel inside, not what you look like outside.** Let's stop making assumptions about other people's identities based on their appearance. Let's stop telling people they can't identify with

being queer if they aren't in a queer relationship. Who you are is something only you know in your heart. How we identify culturally is an attempt to feel more authentic and at home with ourselves, using language that couldn't possibly perfectly illustrate our complexity. The same way what we choose to wear can't. These are just expressions. To really know someone is to know their heart. To really know yourself is to connect to your heart. Trust people when they tell you who they are. They know better than you.

3. **Your gender identity is allowed to evolve.** When I first came out as a teenager I called myself a lesbian. But now that label feels totally off to me, because I don't feel aligned with the category of "woman." It's not like I wasn't a lesbian before — I just kept evolving. And that's okay. We are not stagnant creatures. We are in the process of becoming self-aware. We are unlearning. Let yourself change. Let other people change too.

4. **When someone comes from a different generation than you, in many ways that means a whole different reality.** Making fun of baby boomers is common on TikTok. It's easy to stereotype all people over a certain age as needing to let go of their tired views on gender and sexuality — why is it so hard for them to wrap their heads around gender being a social construct? Well, many in that generation come from an experience where their LHBs about gender were much more ingrained, in which every TV show, every movie, perpetuated those beliefs. For older generations, traditional religion had a much larger influence in the mainstream. That is not an excuse for sexism, homophobia, or transphobia; I'm saying that we shouldn't take for granted the privileges of growing up in the age of the internet. We grew up in a different reality — literally. Keeping that in mind is helpful when you are struggling with having conversations about pronouns with your aunt, who has a lot more years of unlearning to unpack.

5. **It's not feminism unless it's intersectional and trans-inclusive.** Any form of feminism that is hierarchical, whether

that is based on race or gender identity, isn't feminism. The people who want to exclude trans women from feminist circles forget that history has long tried to delegitimize womanhood for various reasons, including behavioral choices, mental capacity, and biological traits. Cis people can transform this bias by calling out exclusionary forms of so-called feminism and defending trans rights.

6. **Another person's experience or relationship to gender does not negate your own.** When you come from an identity that has a history of being marginalized, who you are becomes a badge of honor, and rightly so. The thing is, though, if someone else also identifies that way and comes from a different experience, it doesn't mean that your struggle or hardship matters any less or that their experience is any less legitimate.

    For example, some cis women complain that because a trans woman has never been through an experience like getting her period, she doesn't really know what it's like to be a woman. First of all, not every person with a uterus identifies as a woman, and not every woman with a uterus has an active menstrual cycle. Also, it might be a totally heartbreaking experience for a trans woman not to be able to have a menstrual cycle because everything in her heart aligns with the urge to give birth. The point is, there is no single definition for gender identity, and the difficulties that society has put on people who are socialized as women are also put on trans women in different ways. Again, you are not defined by the limitations of society or hierarchical views.

Affirmations

- My authenticity is my greatest asset.
- I will try to see the Higher Self in others even when they can't see it in themselves.

- I understand another person's inability to support me is a product of their conditioned limitations, not my inadequacies.
- I am not unlovable because someone didn't know how to love me.
- I can trust what my heart is telling me.
- I didn't come out, I let people in.

Journal Prompts

1. The LHBs I grew up with around gender are . . .

2. Those LHBs shaped my self-image by . . .

3. Some challenging experiences I have had around my identity are . . .

4. My Higher Self would respond to those experiences by telling me . . .

5. I am worthy of acceptance and love because . . .

6. The things I love most about myself are . . .

Chapter 15

Mental Health

Me: *I'm so ashamed of my mental health diagnosis. People probably think I'm crazy.*

Higher Self: *The word "crazy" is used to stigmatize mental illness like it's someone's fault they need healing from trauma or are different from the status quo. You are taking care of yourself by getting help, and I'm so proud of you.*

The hospital

As I was walking out of my fifth-period World Geography class, the vice principal of my high school was waiting for me in the hallway. Mrs. Vance was nearly a foot shorter than me, even in her lavender high heels (which perfectly matched her lavender pantsuit). Her signature hair-sprayed brown bob reminded me of a football helmet.

"I need to have a quick chat with you. Follow me," she said.

I thought I must be getting in trouble for too many missed classes. After I moved into Kim's house, we skipped school a lot. Or she might want to talk to me about my run-in with Mrs. Dewitt, my homophobic teacher, who saw me and Kim hugging in the hallway and told us to stop. Maybe she had put in a complaint.

The sound of Mrs. Vance's heels hitting the shiny linoleum flooring reverberated down the hall as I followed her through the back doors of the school to the courtyard, where there were a bunch of portable classrooms beside the teachers' parking lot.

"Let's talk out here so we get some privacy," Mrs. Vance said, without looking at me.

"Okay." *God, I must really be in trouble.*

"So, how are you? How are you doing in your classes?" she asked me as she slowed to a stroll next to me down the sidewalk.

"I'm fine," I said, still confused as to why she'd brought me out here. "Classes are okay."

"I've heard you have been struggling at home. I just want you to know that if you ever need anything, you can come to me." This time she stopped walking.

"Oh, everything is fine at—"

I stopped midsentence as I saw a familiar figure step out of a black car in the teachers' parking lot and start walking toward us.

"Wait...is that my...uncle?"

"Yes, it is," Mrs. Vance said. "He is here to pick you up."

"What? I don't understand."

Then my uncle grabbed my arm and pulled me toward the car.

"You have to come with me now."

Feeling like I had no choice in the matter, I got into the back seat.

"Where are we going? Are my mom and dad okay?" I asked him, still in a state of shock about what was happening.

"Yes, they are fine. We are meeting your mom and dad at your doctor's office."

It took me a minute to realize he was talking about the psychiatrist I had started seeing a couple of months earlier, prompted by a particularly bad fight with my parents. During the fight, I began having a really bad panic attack and couldn't stop crying and screaming, which made my parents get even angrier because they thought I was throwing a fit, like a toddler. They didn't know that I literally could not calm myself down. My dad kept yelling for me to stop, and when I couldn't stop, he said, "Fine, if something is really wrong with you, I'm taking you to the emergency room."

In the hospital parking lot, I begged him not to make me go inside as he tried to drag me from the car while I kicked and screamed. It must have been quite a scene. Eventually I calmed down, and he drove home without me going inside.

When I met Dr. Kay (my psychiatrist), she told me that the reason I had been depressed and having panic attacks was because I had a chemical imbalance in my brain, and that I wasn't making enough serotonin—which she explained is basically a chemical in your brain that makes you happy. For this, she prescribed antidepressants. She told me the pills would likely take weeks to fully work, so I couldn't figure out why I was going back to see her so soon.

My uncle pulled into a parking lot outside a brown brick building I'd never been to before. Inside the automatic doors, it looked like some kind of hospital. My parents were already there, along with Dr. Kay, sitting on a couch by the front desk.

"This is an inpatient treatment center for people your age. Your parents and I both feel that you should stay here for a little bit so you can get the care you need," Dr. Kay said after I sat beside my parents. It had been a week or so since I had seen them, and I never could have imagined it would be in this context.

As she continued talking, it began to dawn on me that this entire scenario had been a setup: My parents and Dr. Kay had been planning on putting me in a mental hospital, and my vice principal had helped conspire to get me outside the school. I was stunned and embarrassed that I hadn't seen it coming.

The irony was, if they had asked me to go, I probably would have. I'd been feeling so depressed that I'd been thinking about dying. Dr. Kay called it "suicidal ideation and morbid thoughts."

I looked over at my parents, who had serious but sad looks on their faces. *Maybe this could be helpful,* I thought. *At least now my parents know I'm not just throwing a fit. At least it looks like they care.*

I agreed to go. After I signed some paperwork, my mom handed me a gift wrapped in pink tissue paper. It was a journal to write in at the hospital, with an angel on the cover. I gave both my parents a hug and a kiss, and Dr. Kay took me past the front desk to my new room.

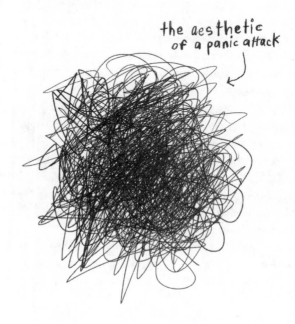

the aesthetic of a panic attack

After being outed at fifteen, I experienced depression for the first time in my life. I had panic attacks and thoughts of suicide, and I was really confused about why those things were happening to me. It felt like I had caught some kind of virus I couldn't fight off.

I knew I was having problems at home, but I was unable to connect feelings of rejection from my parents to my emotional pain and symptoms. My parents wanted me to be at home, but I wouldn't stop seeing my girlfriend. I felt she was the only person who really understood me. I felt like my parents didn't love me. Not the real me. Choosing between coming home or not had become a choice between feeling loved or not.

The treatment center was an inpatient psychiatric hospital for teens twelve to seventeen years old. I was there for two weeks. It was a traumatic experience. The first night I arrived, I listened to another kid bang their head against the wall in the next room for what seemed like hours until staff came in and took the kid away. I cried myself to sleep. They put me on anti-anxiety meds, antipsychotics, and sleeping pills, along with the antidepressants I was already taking.

All of the kids, who were there for reasons that ranged from suicide attempts to sexual trauma, were treated like *they* were the problem. The staff kept order through intimidation. One day, when I refused to comply with a staff member's direction, he threatened me with electric shock treatments if I didn't start behaving (I still don't know if that was a real threat or a fear tactic).

Through good behavior, I earned privileges like going outside or using a plastic fork with my dinner instead of a spoon. We had group therapy every day that felt like a time for confession of everything we had been doing wrong rather than a way to feel better about ourselves.

The entire time I was there, my queerness was never brought up for discussion. I definitely didn't feel safe bringing it up. Neither was the idea that my depression and anxiety might have had something to do with the trauma of being rejected by my parents. There was no discussion about self-love, compassion, or acceptance. It was all about how to change my "behavior problems"—running away from home (even though I felt my parents gave me no choice by saying they didn't allow gay people in the house), taking drugs, and being "uncontrollable."

Later I found out from my parents that my psychiatrist, Dr. Kay (who oversaw my care there), had recommended so forcefully to my parents that I needed to be there, they felt they had no choice. It was a private hospital, not covered by my parents' health insurance and costing tens of thousands of dollars—money that my parents did not have. But they were desperate. They thought they were protecting me. They trusted the doctor. It took them years to pay off that debt.

Connecting to my Higher Self has given me the perspective to look back at this difficult time in my life and see how LHBs about mental illness and cultural LHBs like homophobia impacted my mental health care. My parents, along with many other people in their generation, lacked education and awareness about mental illness as a result of generations of stigmatization, and were terribly unprepared for what was happening to me, with no tools to help. Their homophobia also blinded them from understanding how traumatic it was for me to feel unloved by them. In their minds, there must be something wrong with me, not something wrong with the way they were treating me or something wrong with a society that tells people they should be ashamed of their authentic selves. As a result of homophobia, the doctors and staff at the hospital never addressed the issues at the heart of my trauma. Their approach to my care made me feel like I was the problem, not that I needed help with my problems. What I lacked at that time was love and acceptance. I really needed somebody to tell me, "Hey, you are enough just for being you. There is nothing wrong with you. Let's explore ways we can help you manage these difficult feelings." I needed guidance in accessing the empowerment of my Higher Self—the part of me that knew no matter what my struggles, I was worthy of love, care, and support.

Shame and Stigma

So many of us struggle with our mental health. Some of us in big ways and some of us in small ways. But the biggest misconception about mental health and mental health disabilities is that if you are struggling, there is something fundamentally wrong with you. However, it's easy to feel that way in our culture. The label "crazy"—an extremely unsympathetic characterization that describes a person you should stay away from and who is in some way responsible for their own predicament—is used all the time in TV, movies, and online media. The "crazy" ex-girlfriend, the "crazy" crackhead, the "crazy" ax murderer.

We come from a long history of hierarchical beliefs about mental health problems, mental illness, and trauma. People deemed mentally ill (that term is relatively new; historical labels include "insane," "mad," and "feeble-minded," among others) have been stereotyped, stigmatized, scapegoated, isolated, exiled, imprisoned, abused, tortured, sterilized, used in dangerous experimental surgeries, and condemned to death.

The definition of mental illness and the treatment of people put into this category directly correlates to society's views on what constitutes "normal" behavior, and which hierarchical power structures have a say in those definitions. Which is why a behavior that we would consider normal today—women defending themselves against abuse by their husbands—could have been reason enough for those women to be committed to an insane asylum in the nineteenth century and early twentieth century.

Folks with mental health disabilities—on top of having to manage their illness in a terrible health care system and failing social safety net—face some of the worst forms of social stigmatization and discrimination. A common stereotype is that people diagnosed with serious illnesses such as schizophrenia and bipolar disorder are more likely to be violent, whereas studies show they are no more violent than anyone else, contributing to approximately 4 percent of violent crimes in the United States.

Generations of stigmatization have also prevented people from getting the help they need. Although talk therapy has become more mainstream, there are still so many people who feel too embarrassed or ashamed to seek out that support. They have bought into the narrative that "normal" people should be able to solve their own problems.

Despite the many years of study on the exact causes of mental illness, to this day there is no proven medical cause, only theories. The perception and treatment of mental health disabilities have been influenced by the hierarchical beliefs of those in positions of power. The inequities of society—racism, sexism, homophobia, transphobia, classism, economic disparity, and transgenerational trauma—are still not commonly accepted as important factors in mental health.

With far too little emphasis on society's impact on mental health and way too much responsibility put on the individual, many feel that *they* are the problem. *What's wrong with me?* you ask yourself, which only feeds the negative self-image you are trying to escape. You are depressed about your depression. You are anxious about having anxiety. Layers of shame build up and overwhelm you. Doctors are quick to label their patients as "disordered," with no mention of how a toxic society makes it very difficult to take care of our mental health, or how the cultural stigmatization of mental health struggles might be impacting our self-worth.

You Are Not a Failure

Having a mental health disability or struggling with your mental health is not a personal failure. Having a diagnosis and taking medication does not make you any less valuable, gifted, and lovable. Needing guidance and support to navigate the effects of your trauma just makes you human.

Bringing our Higher Selves to our mental health journey is vital, because we need to distinguish between having problems and the belief that we are a problem.

Our Learned Hierarchical Beliefs often create thoughts in our mind that tell us things like *I'm not good enough* or *I'll never be successful* or *A normal person wouldn't have behaved that way*. But just because we have these thoughts does not make them true. We were conditioned with this perspective. Similarly, the difficult thoughts and feelings we experience when we are struggling with our mental health, whether they are a symptom of PTSD, bipolar disorder, or chronic depression, are also not who we are. They are part of our experience, but they do not define us. In other words, when we awaken to our Higher Selves, we understand that we have always been whole, and the ups and downs of our thoughts and feelings do not diminish that wholeness. It's understandable to feel overwhelmed, embarrassed, or confused when you are going through a difficult time. But it's also important to remember that nothing—good or bad—lasts forever.

Healing Trauma

In a productivity-obsessed culture, we tend to think of healing as a goal to be reached: the harder we work on ourselves, the more healed we will become and eventually our trauma will no longer be an issue. And then when our wounds resurface after we have been working on ourselves, we think we must not be doing a good enough "job" at our healing. But from the Higher Self perspective, healing is a practice, not a goal. It's not about our trauma never showing up in our lives; it's about giving ourselves grace and compassion when it does. Healing is the practice of connecting to your Higher Self, the part of you that knows you are worthy and lovable, the part of you that is the compassionate witness to your struggles, the voice in your heart that says, *I see your struggle and I want you to know that no matter what, you are enough.* Some days that will be easier than others. It doesn't mean you are failing. Sadly, many people believe that until they are fully healed, they are not complete. They use their healing journey as another way to put themselves down. Remember, LHBs are sneaky like that!

My diagnosis

In 2019, I was walking into my therapist's downtown Brooklyn office on a rainy Tuesday afternoon. The room we met in was very small with horrible fluorescent lighting, like a physician's examining room. I'd accepted the less-than-comfortable atmosphere as a trade for sliding-scale pricing — which was the only way I could afford to go.

This particular office catered to a BIPOC queer clientele, and I knew I was lucky to be there. I'd thought about suggesting putting in a lamp in the room to help the ambience, but I was not sure if that was crossing some kind of boundary with my therapist — like criticizing her lighting choices was too personal.

For weeks, I had been struggling — feeling depressed again, probably the worst bout I'd had since being a teenager. Which really surprised me, because everything was going okay in my life. I'd done a lot of healing around my past through my spiritual journey. I was consistently going to therapy. My family was very supportive of me and my relationship. My relationship to art had become so much healthier since I'd begun writing memes about my Higher Self. I'd been unlearning my biased conditioning and working on my body image. In other words, I was doing my "healing work." But the past few weeks, I had found myself inside a tunnel. I felt heavy and dark. At times it felt unbearable, and I couldn't stop crying.

"Hi, Bunny, how was your week?" my therapist asked.

"Um, it was okay. I mean, actually it's been pretty rough."

"Okay. What's been going on?"

"I don't know, just feeling really down, like, how I told you before. Lots of feelings of self-loathing. And sort of like I'm in a tunnel I can't get out of."

"Bunny, I want to tell you that I think you are showing symptoms of major depressive disorder."

The air was sucked out of the room, like when you're trying to blow up a balloon but no matter how hard you exhale nothing seems to come out. All the old feelings of being a scared fifteen-year-old flooded back in. The hospital, the doctors, the feelings of something being fundamentally wrong with me. *Wait, how is this possible? I am a spiritual person. I connect with my Higher Self daily. I've been in therapy for two years. I have major depressive disorder? I am mentally ill?*

My therapist explained that sometimes trauma can live in the body and have physiological effects. And my symptoms, which had lately been really powerful, could be a result of being in a place in my life where I had the space for that stuff to come up.

Although my therapist's words were a bit comforting, I couldn't stop thinking about the fact that I had major depressive *disorder*. I had failed at healing.

For the next few months, I made a conscious effort to ask my Higher Self for guidance around this new "diagnosis." Asking for guidance during my daily meditation had become a practice of mine whenever I was faced with a difficult decision or roadblock. Connecting with my Higher Self helped me see that lessons come in all packages. That even if I was going through something really hard, there was an opportunity to see it through the lens of love. Slowly, I started to become aware of some space between my diagnosis and who I was. That having mental health struggles didn't make me any less spiritual or any less connected to my Higher Self.

Am I mentally ill? On one level of reality, yes. I go through periods of difficult depression. In the past, I would mask it by projecting it on some outside drama; without anything going "wrong" in my life, I no longer had anything to blame these feelings on.

Now when depressive feelings come up, I feel them. And this can last anywhere from a couple of days to the better part of a month. I am working with my therapist on new tools to cope and care for the physiological symptoms.

One thing I have found helpful is to write down messages from my Higher Self and keep them in places I can easily find them — like my desk, my car, my purse, my nightstand. When I am in a depressive episode, these remind me that this moment will pass. I also have other reminders, like a necklace I wear of a white dove. It symbolizes the ethereal nature of my Higher Self, and I hold it when I am feeling down.

The less I identify as a "mentally ill" person, the more I can honor my relationship to that illness, because it lessens its power to make me feel like I am lacking.

We all have difficulties in life, cards we have been dealt that require us to take extra care of ourselves. But our Higher Selves want us to know that those difficulties are just another way we can show ourselves love. And in that way, an "illness" can be a channel for healing.

You're Worthy of Support

Society's understanding of psychological disorders and mental health is constantly evolving. Today you can log on to social media or turn on the news and get an array of explanations for struggles with mental health — from what you eat, to what is happening astrologically, to hormone imbalances, to toxic relationships, to spending too much time online, to not exercising enough or exercising too much.

There are therapists who have different approaches and beliefs, and new studies that contradict what in the past was thought to be common knowledge.

It can be overwhelming and also give you the false impression that if only you figured out exactly what changes you need to make (or what products you need to buy), then you would be healed. But there are a lot of mysteries surrounding the functions of our human-ness. How can we put pressure on ourselves to understand every function of our brains and body when the "experts" are still guessing?

The important thing is that you take the first step of exploring ways you can help yourself. There are many different tools for addressing mental health matters, from psychotherapy to plant medicines to meditation. But no matter what tools work for you, ultimately it's not the method that is most important. The method or tools you use for healing are simply helping you return to the truth that we all share. They are just leading you right back to yourself. It's a journey back home. To the place in you that knows you have always been whole.

Connecting to your Higher Self doesn't mean you will never have mental health struggles; it means you will realize that you are worthy of the care and support you need, even when you are struggling. That you deserve whatever healing tools are out there to support your mental health, and that you are not defined by those struggles—just as your trauma doesn't define you, the ups and downs of your career don't define you, anyone's hierarchical beliefs don't define you.

This world is largely unhealed, and to set ourselves up to a standard of always having to be okay isn't a healthy response. What I realized about my mental illness is that it doesn't make me any less able to tap into my worth, and I need to remind myself that the biggest healing is knowing that at any point in time in my journey, I am enough. There are moments when it's hard to remember that truth. But those moments don't make it any less true.

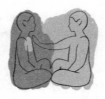

Bring Your Higher Self to Your Mental Health Journey

1. **Stop shaming yourself for the ways you struggle.** Struggling with your mental health in a world that doesn't prioritize mental health or provide equal opportunity for mental health treatment is so understandable! How your brain processes trauma and/or the physiological symptoms you experience is not an indication you aren't worthy of love, kindness, encouragement, and support. Your mental health is an important part of your human experience. Sometimes that experience feels smooth and sometimes it's rough, but who you really are is the *awareness* of that experience. And you can love yourself through it. Shame just adds another unnecessary layer of suffering.

2. **It's okay if it's feeling hard.** Starting a mental health journey is incredibly challenging. Maintaining a mental health journey is hard, too. You're going inward, dredging up the past, and seeing how it shows up in the present. What will sustain you is self-compassion and patience. Your Higher Self is not grading you on your "progress." Your Higher Self just wants you to know you are lovable at every step.

3. **Reach out for help when you need it.** We come from a culture that sees vulnerability as weakness, so it makes sense that many people feel uncomfortable asking for help, especially with their mental health. And so they struggle alone. Sharing your needs is not a weakness; it is a strength, because it means you are strong enough to realize you deserve help. Everyone

deserves support when they need it. If you have been on the fence about reaching out to a therapist or telling a friend that you've been struggling and you need some emotional support to find healing resources, please know that you can and you should. Your Higher Self wants you to. If you are having thoughts of self-harm or suicide, please do not hesitate to call or text 988 for the Suicide and Crisis Lifeline.

4. **Work only with therapists/counselors/healers who make you feel seen and safe.** We all come from different experiences. Which means we will relate to healing styles differently. We will relate to personalities differently. We will even relate to language differently. So it makes sense that some therapists and healers are just not a good match. Likewise, it makes sense that therapists and healers are also people on the healing path, who sometimes make mistakes or are limited in their capacity to empathize or understand issues that are very important to you — like racial trauma or trans identity. Work with people you feel comfortable with. That doesn't mean you won't feel challenged at certain times by the process; it just means you are safe enough with them to be vulnerable.

5. **Utilize additional resources outside of therapy:** Therapy is expensive, and even though there are ways to find therapists who do sliding-scale pricing (definitely check to see if that is available), it's still not *accessible* for everyone. If this is you or you are still looking for a therapist, there are other resources you can use to support your mental health journey. In the Further Reading section of this book I have listed books, podcasts, and social media accounts that I have found very helpful for my mental health journey. There are also free support groups all over the United States that you can attend in person or virtually, and I will list resources for them as well. **Do not ever shame yourself or others for needing medication.** Yes, the pharmaceutical industry is in it for the profit. Yes, the healthcare system needs major reform. But medication is often necessary and saves lives. It pains me to see others in the spiritual

and wellness communities shame folks for using medication as a tool in their healing journey. Everyone deserves the support they need. If you are not sure if medication is for you, the best thing you can do besides working with a therapist (not just a psychiatrist, because they do not spend enough time with you) is to educate yourself about the pros and cons of taking a pharmaceutical approach. Trust your intuition and make a decision from the consciousness of self-worth. Medication is meant to be used in combination with therapy, not in lieu of it.

Reminders

- Stop putting pressure on yourself to have it all together. This world is chaotic. Life is messy. Even nature is unpredictable. So why should you expect to have all the answers? Whatever your best is today, it is enough.
- Whatever you are going through right now is a lesson in accepting yourself. All of yourself. Even the things you are working on changing. There is nothing wrong with you. There never was.
- Beating yourself up is an abuse of power.
- Being hard on yourself feels easy and being easy on yourself feels hard. That doesn't mean you are doing it wrong.
- Today is a good day to tell your past self, "You did the best you could with what you had to work with, and I'm sorry for being overly critical. I love you."
- Shame is not a sustainable form of self-improvement. Stop beating yourself up in order to find the confidence that years of beating yourself up has kept from you.
- Treating your anxiety like an overprotective friend is a much easier way to manage it. It's just trying to keep you safe. So, when your anxiety comes to visit, try letting it know you appreciate the effort, but you are good for right now.

• Sometimes the most toxic relationship you are in is with yourself. Stop putting yourself down. Stop telling yourself you're not good enough. You wouldn't take it from anyone else. So don't take it from yourself.

Writing Exercise

Write a list of your own "Higher Self affirmations" for self-compassion and kindness around your mental health journey. For example, you could write, "I love and accept myself" or "I am loved." There is no right or wrong. When you are finished with your list, incorporate it into your healing practice. Say an affirmation or two when you wake up in the morning. Write one on a Post-it note and put it on your mirror. These affirmations are the voice of your Higher Self, so being able to access that voice, especially on the days it feels hard to hear it, is really helpful. I recommend saying them out loud, not just reading them silently. It makes the message more powerful.

Journal Prompts

1. LHBs that I grew up with about mental health/illness are...

2. The way those LHBs have influenced how I approach my mental health are...

3. Some of my negative thoughts about my mental health are...

4. Flip the script: My Higher Self would respond to each one of those thoughts with...

    _____

5. Changes in my behavior and/or boundaries to better support my mental health journey are...

    _____

6. I deserve love and compassion when I am struggling with my mental health because...

    _____

Chapter 16

Spirituality

Me: *I feel lost. I don't know who I am anymore.*
Higher Self: *No, you are just learning that you are so much more than you thought you were.*

La medicina

At ten o'clock on a Saturday night in 2015, I was sitting in a circle of about fifteen people in a barn in upstate New York. I was so nervous, my palms felt like mini Slip 'n Slides.

Eduardo, the shaman who had traveled from Central America to lead the ceremony, gave us a short talk about the proper etiquette for the night: keeping to our space, not talking to another person during the ceremony, and remembering that we are safe and that he and his helper would be there to guide us. He had an interesting look: a mix between a character from a Carlos Castaneda book and a junior high art teacher.

He then instructed us to approach him one by one for a drink of ayahuasca, starting with the left side of the circle. I made a quick calculation in my mind: *There are six people ahead of me, I probably still have about one minute to back out of this thing. Forty-five seconds, thirty, fifteen, five...now it's my turn.* I knelt down in front of his altar: a blanket on the ground adorned with beautiful flowers, incense, and musical instruments. With a soft but serious face, he poured the dark green liquid into a small cup not much larger than a shot glass and I drank it down. The taste was horrible—like sour-tasting dirt—but I tried not to flinch. I did not want to seem ungrateful.

I went back to my sleeping bag, spread out on a pile of hay. The barn got very quiet as the remainder of the group took their turn. Then the shaman and his helper began to sing icaros and play instruments. It sounded beautiful and strange, and it wasn't long before like their voices and the music completely engulfed me.

I closed my eyes. It felt as though the music had taken me by hand and was leading me down a path of colors and flashes of light, like a slow-motion kaleidoscope. Then I had a vision of myself, but not myself, running down a field. I had a profound sense that I was seeing one of my ancestors on the way to some kind of battle.

Then I was startled by a voice.

"Are you feeling the medicine?"

It was the shaman's helper, Salvador, leaning down in front of me. I realized I'd been in a trance. *How much time has passed?*

"Yes, I think so."

"Do you want some more?"

Yes, I thought. This is very pleasant. This is feeling very good.

"Yes, I would like some more, thank you."

Salvador handed me another drink, this one with noticeably more liquid in it. As the medicine crawled down my throat, it felt like a vine was penetrating my insides until it opened a flower right inside my gut—it was *intense*. I thought to myself, *Oh, I see. This is what all the fuss is about.*

I tried to keep my eyes open, afraid of what might happen if I closed them. But I couldn't do it—something was drawing me into myself, and before I knew it, I was floating in darkness and stars had appeared all around me in blue, red, pink, white...When I focused my eyes on one star, it got bigger and bigger until I was in the star, and within that star were more stars in never-ending fractals. *Is this the meaning of infinity?* Then suddenly I fell, in some kind of a tunnel, down down through space, down down through the clouds, back to the earth, down down through the trees, the leaves, the grass, and into the soil.

Everything was dark. I saw earthworms. Decay. Death. Rot. I got sick to my stomach and threw up in the bucket next to my sleeping bag. I started to panic. I was terrified. I threw up again. I felt so horrible. And I couldn't escape it. It was an awful nightmare. Images of death, pain, darkness, worms. I threw up again. *Should I call for the shaman?* But even speaking felt beyond my capacity. *Am I going to die? Dear God, please help me.*

And then everything went still, and there was a presence with me. A voice said, *There is nothing to be afraid of. Everything is connected. The soil, the stars, you. You are in everything. Everything is in you.* I can only describe this presence as pure love, like all my ancestors holding me with all the compassion and gentleness in the Universe. And then the earthworms came back, but they were pink. They floated into the air and started to dance. They looked like the most perfect little creatures, and I cried realizing how beautiful they actually are. How silly it was for me to be afraid of them. Then I threw up again.

It went on like this for a while. Although I had no concept of time, at moments I felt like I had died and was looking down on my life. I was shown all the people who I loved or had loved me. I saw their smiles, their joy, their pain. I saw their souls and how precious and beautiful each person was: my mom, my dad, my sisters and brother, exes, and friends. I forgave. I let go. I cried, and I purged.

Whenever fear crept in, I purged it out in the bucket. Whenever I got scared, I called out for love and it reappeared. It was a presence. I was held by the greatest feeling of love I had ever felt. It was the most profound spiritual experience I had ever undergone.

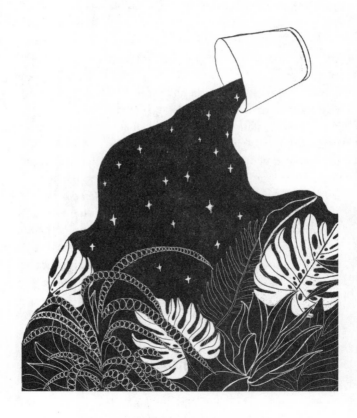

LHBs Masked as Spirituality

My first ayahuasca ceremony was extremely challenging, but I accessed a deeper truth than I had ever experienced. For weeks I felt lighter, more healed, and more tapped into the awareness of love. I decided I would sit for more ceremonies.

However, it wasn't long before I began to unconsciously use my experiences as a way of feeling more "spiritual" than other people. I was spending time in circles of people using plant medicines for healing and spiritual exploration. And a line started to form in my mind between me and my fellow ayahuasca-drinkers, who had seen what I had seen, and everyone else.

My experiences became an identity marker, a way of feeling special, more in tune with the Universe than "most people." I thought I didn't have anything to learn from people who "didn't get it" or who weren't spiritually minded. In fact, I didn't really want to bother being friends with anyone who didn't identify as spiritual.

I also started developing this nagging feeling that I wasn't spiritually advanced enough. I didn't meditate enough, I didn't read enough books, or take enough classes, or sit in enough ceremonies. Sometimes when I meditated, I would shame myself for being distracted, unable to be present. Any time I felt depressed, I blamed it on my lack of spiritual discipline, believing that it was my inadequacy that led to those (weak) feelings. I vacillated between feeling spiritually superior to some and inferior to others.

Most of the Learned Hierarchical Beliefs that we have covered in this book so far have to deal with issues like racism, sexism, and homophobia—issues where those judgmental beliefs (although sometimes unconscious) aren't all that surprising when you shine a light on them.

When it comes to spirituality, those hierarchies are harder to discern, because they are often shrouded in language like "awakened," "evolved," and "aware." But there is no aspect of our life that is immune to hierarchical beliefs. And when it comes to our spiritual path, they can often be sneaky. It's like the "Is it cake?" trend on TikTok, where bakers make cakes that look like inanimate objects. You're scrolling and a video pops up of a knife cutting into a stack of books only to reveal layers of sponge cake and buttercream, and you're like, *Oh, I didn't expect that.* That is what Learned Hierarchical Beliefs packaged in spirituality are—easily disguised, but underneath it's all made of the same stuff.

Our spiritual journeys are a means to awaken to the interconnectedness of all beings, to raise our consciousness to love, and to shift our identity from form to the formless. Some people might define their connection to their Higher Self as their spiritual path. But even if you don't, bringing your LHBs to your awareness is an essential part of your spiritual journey. LHBs either lead you to put yourself down or to put other people down—they are a belief system that keeps you trapped in loveless thinking. They hinder your ability to transcend the limitations of your own bias. They are barriers to compassion. When you approach your spiritual journey from the perspective that you are already whole rather than using it as a means to *make* yourself whole, you don't mistake your spiritual growth as a means to finally feel "good enough." To grow spiritually isn't to become more; it is to realize all that you are.

Working with Spiritual Traditions Outside Your Own

One important way that our spiritual practice is vulnerable to LHBs is when we ignore the cultural lineage of the spiritual traditions we participate in. In *Who Is Wellness For?* the author Fahira Róisín discusses the importance of separating spiritual practices, like meditation and yoga, from the appropriated versions of those practices co-opted by Western capitalism.

She writes, "Part of the obsession of Western confluence with what it interprets as the East's discretion is its incapacity to understand our way of life while totally pilfering it...In order to meditate, you should know the history, and you should also think of why you've never had to think of this before."

It is important to be mindful of the cultural lineage of spiritual practices like yoga, meditation, plant medicine ceremonies, witchcraft, astrology, tarot, acupuncture, and reiki, not only because it is a means of honoring the origins and original practitioners of those traditions, but also to deepen your inner transformation. When you fail to recognize that you are interpreting the meaning of these practices through the lens of your own LHBs, you risk substituting a deeper possibility of healing with an exoticized version, an image of what your LHBs believe it looks like to be spiritual. Spirituality is a means of having a deeper understanding of self, to transcend difficult personal experiences, and to bring more love and peace into your life by connecting to a Divine Source. But many people don't realize how their LHBs steer them away from love and compassion — as was the case with my desire to use ayahuasca ceremonies as a notch on my spiritual résumé, that is, in service to my LHBs. Connecting to my Higher Self brought me back to the awareness of love where I could humble myself with the wisdom that was shared with me and honor it by staying accountable to those lessons. I can feel profoundly grateful for the opportunities to participate in a sacred cultural tradition without taking ownership of it by treating it like spiritual currency, thus appropriating it.

When we use spiritual tools like plant medicines without being mindful and respectful of tradition, we can also end up harming the very thing that has helped us. For example, Western ayahuasca tourism has at the very least a complicated effect on communities in the Amazon. Some anthropologists believe that overharvesting to keep up with demand is putting the medicine at risk of extinction, enabling deforestation and perpetuating the same harm that Indigenous people have faced at the hands of Western capitalism for centuries.

The important thing is to bring awareness to the LHBs that you are working on letting go of and being mindful of the historical and cultural context of your participation in these traditions and rituals. For example, many people participate in a spiritual tradition without thinking about how their own culture has historically oppressed or colonized the very culture that tradition originates from. Being able to recognize that doesn't limit your spirituality; it empowers it because by holding space for that suffering, you expand your capacity for compassion. You honoring that history is an essential part of collective healing. It's imperative to not repeat history and cause more lovelessness in the world. Educate yourself on the historical and cultural lineage of those practices and traditions. Ask yourself what LHBs you are working on letting go of through these practices. This will only make your spiritual practice stronger and more empowered by love.

Our Higher Selves guide us to the heart of our spiritual practice by bringing to light all the barriers to love and compassion in our personal and collective lives. Many contemporary spiritual teachers shy away from talking about issues like politics, ableism, racism, sexism, homophobia, or transphobia. The implication being that those topics aren't "spiritual." But for people whose lives are affected daily by those issues (which I would argue is everyone), these human experiences have a profound effect on their spiritual understanding. Because in order to access compassion within yourself, you need to have compassion for your own painful experiences and the experiences of others. In order to bring more love to the world, you must see where there is lovelessness. LHBs are a system of biases, and it's not enough to call out only the ones that seem to directly impact your life, because in reality they all stem from the same core belief: There will always be a reason we are not good enough. It's the system we have to dismantle. Our journeys are the same.

Holding Space for Suffering

I have often been in spiritual circles where folks are not interested in acknowledging the inequities of the world, and want to keep topics of discussion only on things they perceive as "positive." "Good vibes only" is a common mantra within these groups. They believe that to be spiritual means seeing only love, not pain. Many people now refer to this as toxic positivity or spiritual bypassing.

The spiritual teacher and political activist Marianne Williamson put it plainly when she said, "There is a difference between denial and transcendence." It's understandable to want to steer away from suffering. But there is nothing "negative" about contemplating love-less behavior and/or acknowledging the wounds people carry. It is rather an opening to more love, a doorway to grace. I believe people are afraid to look at suffering not because they don't care but because they don't see how powerful their love is and how much of a difference it makes to people to feel seen by them. You are a blessing to this world and to the people around you. Sharing your compassion, holding space for other people's pain, is a spiritual strength, an affirmation of the profound love in your heart. It also reminds you of how resilient your spirit is—that often in our darkest moments, we can have the most profound spiritual insight. As the mystic poet Rumi said, "Suffering is a gift. In it is hidden mercy."

In his autobiography, *Being Ram Dass,* which was published after his passing in 2019, Dass (a white man) tells a story about leading a retreat on spirituality and activism in the early nineties. During the retreat, his lectures on meditation did not go over well for the activists in the group, who were largely people of color. How could this white man who had little understanding of their experience lecture them on "how they should see things"? He says, "It soon became apparent how difficult it is to be silent (in meditation) unless you feel that your voice has been heard." The experience was a spiritual insight that he didn't realize he needed. Becoming aware of the historical and cultural context his participation represented to other people in the group didn't hinder spiritual connection; it expanded the capacity for deeper understanding and compassion.

Every one of us carries our LHBs, our trauma, and our past experiences with us. They can be a hindrance to our spiritual growth or they can be openings to deeper truths, depending on the consciousness with which we use them. With the awareness of your Higher Self, they become portals to more love, compassion, and connectedness.

There Is No One Way to Be Spiritual

When I use the term "spirituality," I use it inclusively as an umbrella term for any tradition or practice that opens you up to a Divine Source within yourself, including religion. There is no hierarchy within the various teachings that exist in the world, only what best serves you and your beliefs. In contemporary spiritual circles there can be a tendency to judge organized religion as a less enlightened path because of the way it has been used in service to patriarchal, homophobic, and transphobic LHBs. However, as mentioned before, LHBs can and do show up in nonreligious spiritual practices. What is important is to distinguish the difference between the teachings of love and the hierarchical lens those teachings are unfortunately interpreted through. The moment we start judging one practice as being better than the other, or one person as being more spiritual than the other, we fall into hierarchical thinking. When all paths lead to love, there is no wrong path. When everyone is a spirit being, no one can be more or less spiritual.

From the Higher Self perspective, spirituality isn't about reaching some destination or some mountaintop where you can look down on others and feel like you've "made it." It's about realizing that you are whole *right now* in this present moment; it's about recognizing that wholeness in all beings. Each one of us is an embodiment of love. No matter what we have been through or where we come from. That love is a radiant light that shines from within and touches everything it comes in contact with. It is our greatest gift. It is a gift that will transform the world. Don't limit your light. The world needs it.

Spirituality is the most empowering yet humbling path. Empowering because you realize how worthy you are, and humbling because you realize that everyone else is worthy, too.

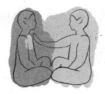

Bring Your Higher Self to Your Spirituality

1. **Toxic positivity and spiritual bypassing are two oxymorons.** There is nothing positive or spiritual about denying the suffering of others. Remember, the essence of spirituality is love, and sometimes the best spiritual support you can give someone is to validate their suffering and show them compassion. This is the essential first step before offering another way of seeing the situation or another perspective inspired by your spiritual understanding and experience.

2. **Your spiritual path is not going to be the same as everyone else's, and that is a good thing.** There are many different traditions, practices, rituals, and teachers out there. No single path has a monopoly on truth. We all relate to language and environment differently. We all come from different experiences. So it makes sense that what might work for me doesn't work for you. Or that some practice might have helped you in the past, but now you want something different. The "practice" isn't the point. It is an arrow pointing you to the same truth that all practices do. To your wholeness and connection to all creation.

3. **Don't make assumptions about what it looks like to be spiritual or on the path of enlightenment.** When I first started dating my spouse, I was concerned that we wouldn't be compatible because they didn't identify as "spiritual." They didn't have any crystals (I slept with a rose quartz under my pillow every night), and they didn't do yoga or meditate. But soon I began to see how spiritual they were, even if they didn't call it

that. They went on long walks in nature alone, had a deep relationship to their plants and art, and could access a profound inner peace that was so beautiful to witness. I realized how spiritually inspiring they were. There are many portals to the Divine.

4. **Thinking of your Higher Self as a spiritual concept is wonderful, but it's okay if you don't.** We all relate to spirituality differently. We all relate to love differently. If you look up the definition of spirituality, you will get a wide range, from religious tradition to esoteric teachings to just a path of inner peace. The purpose of this book is to connect you to the state of consciousness where you are aware of your wholeness, your value, and your inherent connection to all Creation because you are a part of Creation. I use the term "Higher Self," "Higher" implying a higher state of awareness/consciousness. But ultimately the language is not nearly as important as what is in your heart. So if you define your Higher Self as your spiritual awareness, that's beautiful. If you define it as a psychological shift in perspective or a philosophical way of approaching life, that's beautiful too! It's all about unlearning in order to find your truth.

Meditation for Accessing Your Higher Self

Find a quiet place where you will not be disturbed. Set a timer on your phone for fifteen minutes. Sit upright in a comfortable position. Close your eyes and begin focusing on your breath. Imagine there is a bright light in the area of your chest where your heart is. It is glowing. It feels warm and safe. Your whole body is relaxed, comforted by this warm light. This light is your Higher Self. It has always been there and always will be. It is the light of love. Now internally say these words: "I am a representative of love. I am my Higher Self." Repeat these words while continuing to breathe calmly until the timer goes off.

Journal Prompts

1.   LHBs that I carry with me about spirituality are...

2.   The biggest hindrance to my spiritual growth is...

3.   Flip the script: What would your Higher Self say about your perceived hindrance?

4.   Changes in my behavior and/or boundaries I can implement to support my relationship to spirituality are...

5.   New ways I'm interested in expanding my spiritual understanding are...

6.   Things I can do every day to reconnect with my spirit are...

7.   My Higher Self is divine because...

Chapter 17

Self-Care

> **Me:** *Life is hard.*
> **Higher Self:** *So maybe you should stop being so hard on yourself.*

Burned out

It was five thirty a.m. and still dark outside when the alarm on my phone went off. Khara and our dog, Rio, were sound asleep, and I tried to ignore the ping of resentment. My body felt like it was moving through Jell-O as I slowly sat up and headed to the bathroom to pee.

For months, I had been having trouble staying asleep. When I'd first go to bed, I would pass out, exhausted, but then I would wake up around two a.m., jolted by a thought of something I should have done or a worry about something in the future. I'd lie there for hours, anxious. Sometimes I'd get on my phone and scroll to silence my thoughts. Then it took me an hour or two to doze off again. By the time I got to bed the next night,

I'd fall asleep right away, exhausted, and the cycle would continue.

I began setting my alarm a couple of hours earlier than usual after I started writing this book. I figured the only way I was going to get it done while still working on all my other projects and deadlines was to carve out extra hours in the morning.

Before this whole book thing, I used to wake around seven or eight a.m. and leisurely perform my morning self-care routine: meditation and journaling. It was one of my favorite times of the day—sitting in my living room, copal or sage filling the air, feeling the warmth of the new morning sun on my cheeks while meditating. I'd pour my first cup of hot coffee and write all my feelings and reflections in my journal while I sipped it down. Even if I woke up feeling crappy, by the time I finished journaling, I'd have channeled into my Higher Self and my perspective would have shifted.

But with the book, my self-care routine changed. I was so afraid that I wouldn't meet my deadline that I figured working on it for a few more hours a day was a better form of self-care than meditation and journaling; at least this way I wouldn't be stressed about not getting the work done. In other words, I was working more to de-stress. But my plan wasn't working. No matter how much I got done, it was never enough to calm me down. I was in some sort of relay race where one stressful thought led to another, except all the team members were me and I never got to the finish line.

Our wooden staircase creaked as loudly as you might expect in a house that was built in the 1880s as I headed to the kitchen to feed the cats and make coffee before I got to writing.

Right on schedule, Pepper and Zoro began their meowing countdown, weaving in and out of my legs like synchronized swimmers, a routine that would not stop until they were fed.

"God dammit," I said out loud when some of the juice from their "chicken liver feast" got on my hand. As I washed it off in the sink, a realization popped into my head, like the theme music from an old sitcom.

Oh fuck, I forgot to get coffee yesterday! We don't have any coffee!

The thought that I wasn't going to have any caffeine to fuel the thousand words I had promised myself I would finish before eight a.m., the gnarly Fancy Feast mystery meat liquid that smells like Vienna sausages dripping onto the sleeve of my robe, and the exhaustion I felt from so many days in a row of not getting a full night's sleep, combined with the impending doom of my book deadline, was too much for me to hold.

I broke down and started bawling so hard that I could no longer stand and just plopped down on the kitchen floor. "I can't do this!" I said to myself through tears. "I can't write a book. I can't sleep. I can't do anything! I'm such a failure!" Outside my window I saw a neighbor pass by walking their dog, illuminated by the streetlight. Their gaze turned toward my kitchen as if they could sense me looking at them. *Oh God, did he just see me crying on the kitchen floor, like a toddler having a tantrum?* I felt humiliated. Meanwhile the cats continued to meow.

Higher Self-Care

Learned Hierarchical Beliefs put pressure on all of us in different areas of our lives — whether that is to be the best mom we can be, or the best artist, or the best entrepreneur; to fit into a certain dress size; to be the perfect husband; to meet our parents' expectations; or to make all of our friends happy.

We have all been brought up to feel like we have to earn our self-worth. From that lens, self-care is seen as a reward we can give ourselves only after we have worked hard enough on something that will be in service to our LHBs. Usually, this is a way to fit into an image of what we are told success, happiness, and health look like, even if the goal in question does nothing to improve our actual well-being.

For example, exercise can be a great form of self-care, but many people exercise to fit into a body image they feel will make them worthy. Every time they work out, they judge their bodies, bouncing up and down on the LHB roller coaster of feeling confident one day and inadequate the next, depending on the number on a scale or the reflection in the mirror.

Or some people might take themselves on a shopping spree as a form of self-care, even if it puts them in a financially vulnerable position, or use it as a distraction from difficult feelings they might need to address.

My twisted logic of sacrificing my morning meditation and journaling and replacing it with the "self-care" of working more to "gain confidence" only added to the belief that unless I did more, I wasn't deserving of care. Which fed into my conditioned fears of not being good enough, adding more pressure to my career accomplishments to fulfill my sense of lack. This inevitably made the work less enjoyable and more difficult.

It seems like everywhere on social media, people are talking about self-care. Even companies advertising skin cream or hair products position them as something you should buy for your "self-care routine." And it makes sense that companies are targeting their audiences with this type of marketing. Our world seems to be more chaotic every day. Many people are struggling with feeling healthy and happy. We are overworked, juggling multiple responsibilities, taking care of loved ones, and struggling to pay bills. We scroll on our phones to try to wind down, only to get overstimulated by the endless images, videos, news stories, and latest social media drama.

Trying the latest self-care product or trend can help you feel like you are doing something to improve your well-being. But ultimately none of these products, trends, or practices will work if you are not conscious of what the purpose of self-care really is.

What I am talking about is the difference between so-called self-care in service to our LHBs that keep us trapped in the lens of inadequacy, and self-care from your Higher Self perspective — which I will call Higher Self–care.

Higher Self–care isn't only rewarding yourself for meeting your goals or taking action to try to fit into some predetermined concept of what self-improvement looks like; **Higher Self–care is any behavior or practice that reminds you of your fundamental truth:** You are already enough and you always have been.

Higher Self–care is less about the form it takes and more about the intention behind it. Form is what you do for self-care and how often you do it. Intention is *why* you do it. Are you doing it to connect to the part of you that knows you are worthy of rest, joy, and peace, or are you doing it because your LHBs tell you in order to be enough you need to do *more*? Unless we are connected to our worth, we actually won't be in touch with what choices to make that will best serve us. How many of us have put ourselves down for not going to a yoga class we've been meaning to go to when the whole point of yoga is to be in touch with our wholeness, not to add it to our to-do list of things we must accomplish in order to like ourselves so when we miss it, yoga becomes a tool to beat ourselves up with. Our Higher Selves help us remember that no matter what, we are enough, and not doing something on your self-care list doesn't mean you've failed at caring for yourself. Giving yourself grace is one of the most important ways you can care for yourself.

Every human on this planet experiences stress to varying degrees. Because this world is stressful! But what we often don't acknowledge is the invisible layer of stress we put on ourselves when we are afraid that any inability to meet our goals is an indication of how worthy we are or how much we deserve.

As we covered in previous chapters, there are many things about how our world functions that are not equal, are unjust, and need to change — this is because so much of our lives is organized around LHBs, the belief that some people are more deserving than others. But none of that change is possible on a systemic level until we acknowledge how our own internalized LHBs have convinced us that we are unworthy, and realize the harm that belief has caused and continues to cause. In so many circumstances we unconsciously oppress ourselves, denying ourselves rest, nurturing, leisure, pleasure, and joy just for being who we are. Because on a fundamental level we don't realize we deserve it.

No More Self-Harm in the Name of Self-Care

If we are not conscious of how our LHBs influence our choices around self-care, even our self-care routines can be a vehicle for putting ourselves down. After I realized that sacrificing my morning meditation and journaling for more work wasn't helping me be less stressed or even more productive, I went into a shame spiral. Here I was trying to write a book about how to connect with your Higher Self, and I was doing such a shitty job at connecting with mine. Not only was I failing at writing, but now I was failing at my self-care. Double failure!

Do you see how sneaky LHBs can be? That we can use even the ways in which we are trying to take care of ourselves to put ourselves down? When we are stuck in the consciousness of our LHBs, nothing we do will ever be good enough.

Your Higher Self is not interested in shaming or guilting you to take care of yourself. All that does is keep you in the mental trap of low self-worth that led you to sacrifice your well-being in the first place. Your Higher Self is a voice of compassion, acceptance, and encouragement, and will always be there to remind you that no matter what choices you have made in the past, **you can always choose self-love now**. No matter what chaos is happening in the world, you deserve inner peace. We all do.

So the next time your to-do list is overwhelming you and you think the last thing you have time for is a thirty-minute meditation or yoga class or even a nap, tell yourself, "No matter how much I get done on this to-do list, I am enough." I can't tell you the number of days that saying that to myself would have made a difference. We so rarely give ourselves that love and care. But we need it so badly. Life is hard, so we need to stop being so hard on ourselves.

Self-Care Is Not Conditional

A couple of months into the pandemic lockdown in NYC, Khara and I had left our Brooklyn apartment only a few times to get food and supplies. Every morning, we'd wake up and look at our phones to check the latest number of Covid cases and read the news: stories of people who had lost family members, the hospitals becoming full to capacity with dwindling numbers of ventilators, and families that weren't able to have a funeral in person or grieve together.

We'd lie in bed at night and listen to the sounds of ambulances every five minutes. We were always worried, imagining what would happen if we got sick or our family did. What if they never found a vaccine? Would things ever return to normal? It all felt like too much to hold. Too much sadness and too much fear. I couldn't bear it.

In the past when I'd feel overwhelmed, I'd go to yoga or the gym, or meet up with my best friend for a walk in Prospect Park to decompress. But all of that was gone. Even going on a walk felt risky. This was right in the beginning of mask recommendations — the stage where everyone was washing their groceries. On the news they said the best way to protect yourself and others was to stay home (if you were privileged enough to do that).

Trying to get us out of our slump, Khara suggested I find some new form of self-care I could do at home, something to take my mind off the pandemic, like a craft project. They had just started making a hand-sewn quilt. They'd sit on the rug in our living room and cut out square patches of fabric with the focus of an eight-year-old working on their favorite Lego set.

"What about that embroidery kit I got you last year for Christmas?" they suggested.

But a craft project to take my mind off the pandemic felt wrong, like I was ignoring the pain of others. I didn't want to distract myself. *How does it make sense that there are people out there dying alone or risking their lives to make sure we have groceries, and I can sit here safe on my couch thinking of some new creative project for self-care?* It felt selfish and absurd.

But scrolling on social media, reading the news, and posting my memes on Instagram could fill only so many hours a day, and reluctantly I took out the embroidery kit collecting dust on the top shelf of my closet.

At first it was incredibly frustrating. I kept messing up threading the tiny eye of the needle. I watched some YouTube videos on embroidery technique: *Needle in…pull…needle in…pull…* each strand of thread filling in a space no wider than a few millimeters thick.

It struck me how long it had been since I'd made anything creative that didn't have to do with my "career." I couldn't even remember. *Needle in…pull…needle in…pull….* I was used to making something and immediately posting it on Instagram. But this project was going to take a long time, and there was no audience to show it to. No likes to count… *needle in…pull…needle in pull…* The repetition was slowing my breathing and then my heart… For the first time in weeks, I started to soothe.

As I stitched, I realized that embroidery as a form of self-care wasn't about distracting myself at all. It was an intentional time to slow down my thinking, to be present in the repetition, to not make it about success or being "good" at something. To just be with myself in the moment, and let that be enough.

I realized that constantly obsessing about the news was distracting me from a deeper truth about the pandemic: We all deserve care, and denying myself care in the face of suffering wasn't serving anyone. It certainly wasn't helping me connect to my Higher Self, the part of me that knows my own value and enables me to see the value in all people.

Life is precious and beautiful and fragile. We are all just threads being pulled in this direction and that, and if we don't take time to slow down, we can miss the big picture.

Higher Self–care is about nurturing intimacy with yourself so you can tune in to what you really need, what is really important, and the peace you deserve. It can come in many forms—going on a walk, meditation, painting your toenails, taking bubble baths, or literally doing nothing at all.

We tend to think of self-care the way the wellness industry sells it to us, things like eating only organic foods, a massage treatment, buying a product that will improve you in some way, or going on a five-day yoga retreat.

Of course, all of those things can be amazing forms of self-care. But what we often miss is that self-care doesn't have to come in big packages or cost money. And spending money on self-care products won't necessarily help you connect to your self-worth.

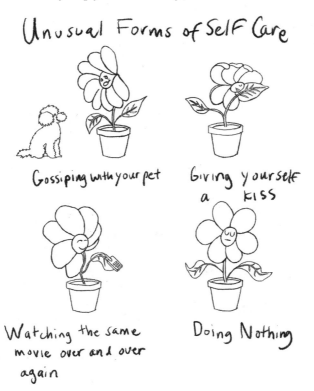

Unusual Forms of Self Care

Gossiping with your pet

Giving yourself a kiss

Watching the same movie over and over again

Doing Nothing

The greatest form of self-care is treating yourself with care. Saying nice things to yourself. Giving yourself encouragement and reminders of how worthy you are and how much you deserve.

Higher Self–care is focusing on nourishing your self-worth and acknowledging that you have always been enough. These are the most important ways you can care for yourself—behaviors that remind you of that truth.

If you are not used to that, it can feel awkward, uncomfortable, even selfish. If the people around you aren't used to you prioritizing your self-care, it can also catch them off-guard.

Some people have said to me, "I don't know how to self-care." To which I reply, "I don't believe you. You care for people every day. You take care of your loved ones. You are sympathetic to your friends' struggles and try to make them feel better. You know exactly how to love and care for someone. Don't you think you deserve that as well?"

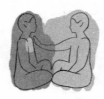

Bring Your Higher Self to Self-Care

1. **Remember, it's less about what you do, and more about the intention behind it.** Try to be mindful of what your self-care is in service to. Why are you meditating? Because if you don't you will feel ashamed of yourself? Or because it genuinely helps you? Why are you going to that Zumba class? Because you're in a spiral of fatphobia? Or because it helps you connect

to your body and feel more powerful? Sometimes it just takes a quick check-in before you do it. All you have to do is remind yourself of your Higher Self intention. And it will make it even more relaxing and nourishing, I promise!

2. **When you don't have time for anything else, you have time to say nice things to yourself.** I get it. Some days even taking a bubble bath just feels like another thing "to do." Some days, there's barely time to go pee. (Hello, moms of young kids or restaurant workers on an eight-hour shift.) But getting in the routine of saying sweet things to yourself — that is, using your Higher Self voice — makes a huge difference, especially in the mornings, because it helps set the tone for the day.

3. **Don't be afraid to try new things.** I honestly don't think we get curious enough about trying new things that could bring us joy or pleasure. We just aren't used to it. But what if joy was your priority in life? What if it became number one on your list? What would change if you ventured outside what you know? What would you do differently? What would you experiment with? What are you waiting for?

Reminders

- Today is a good day to not let your capitalist conditioning equate self-compassion and rest with complacency and insufficient productivity.
- You were conditioned to believe that in order to be deserving, you need to be struggling. What you call hard work is really you being too hard on yourself about your work.
- Whatever you are doing right now would be easier if you were being nice to yourself.
- Being a people pleaser is no excuse for not taking care of yourself, because aren't you also a person who deserves to be pleased?

- Loving yourself isn't hard. Accepting that you love yourself is hard because then you'd have to treat yourself better. Loving yourself isn't about you changing, it's about your behavior changing.
- You have always been your "best self." You are just in the process of changing your perception of that truth.

Journal Prompts

1. LHBs that I carry with me when it comes to my relationship to self-care and rest are...

2. I got those LHBs from...

3. Flip the script: My Higher Self would say this about my self-care and rest...

4. Changes in my behavior and boundaries that would support my self-care are...

5. Ways that I can care for myself that I never thought of before are...

6. I am proud of myself because...

7. When I feel at peace with myself I am doing...

_____

8. Examples of ways I could be nicer to myself throughout my day are...

_____

Chapter 18

Higher Purpose and "Finding Your Passion"

> **Me:** *I wanna be my best self.*
> **Higher Self:** *You already are. You are just strengthening your perception of that truth one day at a time.*

Your Passion Is What You Love to Do, Not What You Do in Order to Love Yourself

There is a lot of rhetoric out there about finding your passion — that one thing you are meant to do in the world. I believe that we all have a role to fill in the awakening of love on the planet. I believe that fulfilling that role is necessary for our human species to survive, take care of our shared home, and create a safe and loving future for generations to come.

I think often when we talk about passion, people see it through a hierarchical lens. If a person doesn't know what their passion is, they feel incomplete. Or if what they spend most of their time doing isn't something they see as "special" or "unique" or something they think will save the world, they feel they are lacking some fundamental part of themselves. Or if their passion isn't paying their bills, they feel they are failing.

I want to illustrate the difference between a passion and a higher purpose. A passion is something you love to do, that brings you joy. This can evolve. It's not something you choose one day and then have to do for the rest of your life. For example, for years your passion might be to be a mom, or to get your graduate degree, or to do tarot readings. And then later it might become something else, or multiple things at a time. Or you might be in a transition where you are not yet sure what you are passionate about. And that happens. There is nothing wrong with that.

Following your passion is often not easy, especially if expectations were put on you to have a certain career or have three kids by the time you are thirty. There is also a lot of cultural bias about pursuing something outside the box, like non-Western healing practices, or starting your own business reading birth charts, or selling your crafts on Etsy.

Your higher purpose, however, never changes and is the same as everyone else's higher purpose—to bring more love into this world by awakening that love within yourself. Your higher purpose informs *everything* you do: From the things you enjoy to the things you don't enjoy. From intimate relationships to art projects. From throwing a birthday party to cooking a meal. You are here on this planet in this human form to take part in a collective shift in our shared consciousness.

Every morning you wake up, you have a choice. That choice is to go about your day willing to see love in all situations, as a representative of your Higher Self—the awareness of how worthy you are and how worthy everyone else is, or to act in the world unconscious of love. To let LHBs run your life and to refuse to be accountable.

Your higher purpose is the path of love. Passion is what you do, and your higher purpose is stepping up to the responsibility that what you do is secondary to the state of consciousness with which you do it.

Discovering my true purpose

I feel grateful that I have always known what my passion is. I am an artist. I have been since I was little. I'm a sucker for making my creative ideas come to life. I love performing, writing, and making visual art. Hell, I even enjoy making TikToks.

But one day I woke up and realized that my passion wasn't my higher purpose. It's just one of the forms through which that purpose is expressed.

A couple of weeks after I started posting my Higher Self memes on Instagram, I logged on to the app and noticed something that made me gasp out loud. Chani Nicholas had liked a couple of my memes and was now following me.

Chani Nicholas was my new favorite astrologer. Since I'd been on a mental health break from posting my art and trying to take care of myself, I decided to sign up for one of her online workshops about the second and tenth houses in astrology. These houses are about your assets and your career. I thought it might be helpful, considering I was at this time in my life when I had no idea what was happening with my music and art career, and the only thing I could do was make memes about just trying to be okay in the world.

When I took the workshop, I expected my birth chart to reveal that my career was supposed to be about performing, but what stuck out to me was that my tenth house is in Cancer, typically indicative of a nurturing role or emotional healing. Something in me was like, *Huh, healing*. I took it as a sign to keep making the memes. So when I saw Chani was following me just a short time later, it felt like more than a coincidence.

Later that day at my job waiting tables, I told one of my coworkers the story about how I took the astrology workshop from Chani on a whim, kept making the memes, and now, out of nowhere, she was following me.

"You should DM her and tell her that," my coworker said to me.

"Oh, I don't think I can," I replied.

"Why not?!"

"I'm just shy, I don't know. What if she thinks I'm bothering her?"

"Babe, trust me, if her work is helping people, she would want to know. Wouldn't you?"

That night when I got home, I reluctantly opened the app to Chani's page and hit the message button.

> Hi Chani! Just wanted to reach out cus I saw you liked my Higher Self meme and you directly inspired me to make them! I took your 2nd/10th house workshop and learned about my assets. Then when I saw you liked one I just had to tell you how full circle that was for me. You're a big inspiration, keep doing what you are doing!

Chani replied:

> OMGSS!! I love your posts! You have an amazing aesthetic sense. What's your Libra situation?

My sun, rising, Venus, Mercury, Saturn, and Pluto are all in Libra in my birth chart. Chani knows her stuff! I had a deep sense that I was being guided by something bigger than myself—bigger than a career.

Soon after my conversation with Chani, I went to my desk, took out a piece of paper, and wrote this down:

What Do People Need Now?

1. Freedom to be themselves (a safe space)
2. Inspiration to contribute to humanity
3. A unique voice/self-expression
4. To feel loved, respected, and appreciated
5. To heal from past trauma

How can I help?

I decided right then that I would only share publicly if what I was sharing fit into one of those categories. That paper is now framed on the wall at my office.

It wasn't the form of the message that was the most important; it was the intention behind it. It wasn't about being cool or better than other people. It wasn't about being famous or proving I was gifted. It wasn't even about the art. It was the *purpose* of it. That was what needed to shift. The purpose of my work is love. Until I realized that, I was blocking the love my work was trying to give me!

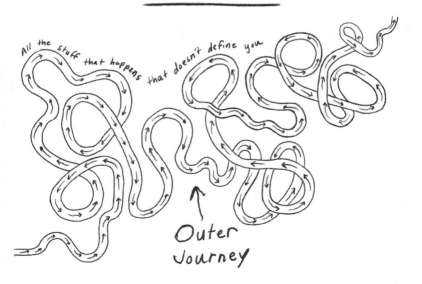

The Path of Love

The reason why the state of your consciousness is so important is because it is connected to our collective human consciousness. And when you shift to the awareness of love, you are participating in our collective awakening.

In order for our world to change, it's going to take a lot of action on our part, but that action cannot be healing or transformative unless its intention is love. **It is imperative to stay focused on your higher purpose and to let love guide your path.**

Now you might be reading this and saying, *Okay, but I still want to know what my passion is. I still want to succeed in fulfilling my dreams and doing what I love.*

To which I will remind you that in order to truly do what you love, you have to be in the consciousness of love. I spent years making art, but so much of that time was spent in the consciousness of fear, insecurity, and despair. When you are in the consciousness of love, you see how every experience you have and have had is a curriculum to your awakening. When you are in the consciousness of love, you let your Higher Self guide your choices.

That might mean making drastic changes to your job or your environment, doing something you have always been afraid to do; it might mean doing the same thing you've done every day, but realizing that you need to show up differently. In every space you walk into, you are a representative of love.

Dharma, a philosophical concept derived from spiritual traditions including Hinduism and Buddhism, has been generalized to Western audiences by popular spiritual teachers such as Deepak Chopra and Sahara Rose to mean aligning with your soul's purpose. Everyone has a dharma based on their talents, gifts, and the wisdom of their experiences, and they can use them to help create a better world.

I absolutely agree. I believe that we all have a unique way of sharing our wisdom and creativity, and that we can all contribute to change.

I think the danger, however, is that so much of Western hierarchical thinking can take a beautiful concept like dharma and turn it into just another way of not feeling good enough, leading to the feeling that unless you find your dharma or life's purpose, you are not complete. You are not doing enough. So you anxiously take the "dharma" quiz online or sign up for that workshop. *I'm not living my dharma! I gotta hurry up and find out what my dharma is! It needs to be something big! Something super impactful!* And it just becomes another thing you believe will finally make you whole. You might even feel more evolved than other people because your dharma is "better" than someone else's. Or more glamorous. Or more successful. Remember, Learned Hierarchical Beliefs are so sneaky!

Focusing on your state of consciousness and the realization that you have always been enough is essential. From that place, you engage with the world with an open heart, seeing opportunity to love in even the unlikeliest of places. We rarely realize how even the smallest acts of kindness can drastically change someone's life. Aligning with your higher purpose isn't about figuring out the one thing you are supposed to do (although for some people there will be one point of focus where they contribute most of their energy), it's about showing up for love in all parts of your life.

Becoming a painter and working on art for eight hours every day is a beautiful contribution to this planet, and you may see painting as your dharma. But if you're stuck in a cycle of toxic behavior once you come home from the art studio, are abusive in your relationships, or abusive to yourself, you are not embodying your Higher Self; and as much as painting is a positive contribution to our collective consciousness, it is often diminished by the harm in other parts of your life.

I think that is why it's hard when a really talented artist or someone we have really admired is revealed to have a personal life that is disappointing or even abusive. We think, *How could someone with so many gifts and talents who has put so much beauty in this world also have caused so much harm?* Because love isn't just about what we do; it's understanding who we are. When we know we are love, we see that every part of our lives is interconnected. We don't compart-mentalize our healing.

Today I have to be extra mindful that my LHBs and fears of inadequacy don't filter into the work I do, that I don't use my plat-form in service to my hierarchical desires. The truth is, I know it's possible to be both helping people and harming myself at the same time. I can put out a podcast episode or a post on Instagram with the greatest intentions to help people, and then come home at night and beat myself up. My higher purpose is beyond the work I put into the world, although that is a big part of it—it's a commitment to love. To love myself and to love you. Of course, I won't always get it right. This path is not easy.

You and I are on the same journey. Back to ourselves. Back to the realization of our Oneness with each other. Back to home. To our hearts. To honor the Higher Self in all beings. To be present in the beauty of this magnificent planet. To know in every part of our mind, body, and spirit that we deserve abundance, safety, nurtur-ing, and peace. We have always been enough, and we are part of creation, united in love.

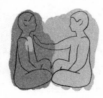

Align with Your Higher Purpose

1. **Don't get caught up in judging whether other people are aligning with their higher purpose.** You don't know their journey or what form the curriculum of their healing should

take. All you can do is be diligent about your perspective, your journey, and showing up with love. We can't control people's choices. But we can inspire them by showing them how valuable they are. The best form of teaching is to demonstrate. Trust in your Higher Self and you will naturally help others trust in theirs as well.

2. **You are allowed to make mistakes, to change your mind, and to not know what you want.** Do not put pressure on yourself to have all the answers. Mistakes are how we learn. Lots of stuff is trial and error. Your Higher Self is compassionate and patient and wants you to just take things one day, one thought at a time.

3. **All you have to be is yourself.** You were created whole, a gift to this world. You are enough. The best part about you is there is no other you. So why would you try to be anything but yourself?

4. **Everything you have been through in your life has brought you here right now—an amazing place to be.** You are wise. You are strong. You are courageous. Do not play small. Do not hinder your light. Radiate. Shine. Nothing is holding you back. Everything is pushing you toward love. Allow it to happen. Let go and surrender to your truth. You are your Higher Self.

Reminders

- Sometimes your goals have to take a back seat to healing and tending to your spirit. It doesn't mean you won't get there; it means when you get there, you will be ready. Often your insecurity is actually the process of unlearning dependence on outside validation. You are on the verge of real security—the kind that says, "I don't need anyone's permission to love myself."
- Impostor syndrome is a precursor to realizing you are here to disrupt and revolutionize the status quo.

- Your predictions about the future are reimagined experiences of the past because that is all you know. In truth, the future contains all possibilities.
- There is no such thing as rejection; there is only the Universe saying, "You are meant for something else."
- You are not lost. You are evolving, so your surroundings are going to seem unfamiliar.
- Stop waiting for permission to feel worthy. Stop waiting for the relationship, the body image, the success, or the people who have hurt you to change. You give yourself permission. You are what you have been waiting for.
- Contraction is a natural part of growth. If you don't think things are happening for you fast enough, maybe the lesson is that you are already enough. Maybe that is the growth that really matters.

Journal Prompts

1. Ways I've used the pursuit of my passion to put myself down are...

   _____

2. Things I love to do and why are...

   _____

3. I can share more love in the world by doing little things and big things like...

   _____

4. I can show myself more love by...

   _____

5. Things I'm interested in doing or learning about for the first time are...

6. I can get out of my comfort zone because...

7. My Higher Self defines my passion and purpose as...

A Note Before We Say Goodbye

We are on the same journey. Like you, I am awakening to my Higher Self. I am unlearning every day. Sometimes I want to throw in the towel. Sometimes the world feels like just too much. Sometimes relationships are so freaking hard. But then I take a deep breath and remember love is who I really am and who you really are. No matter what we face in the future, nothing can take away the love that is our greatest power. I see you. And I am so proud of us. We got this.

I love you and so does your Higher Self.

Bunny

Acknowledgments

When I first decided I wanted to write a book I knew it was going to be hard, but what I didn't fully understand was that I wasn't going to do it alone. What an honor this has been.

First, I would like to thank my mom, Peta, my dad, Marcos, and my sisters, Felili and Maria, for graciously supporting me narrating my personal experience in our shared history. I know people will feel seen in our stories, and it has been such a gift to collaborate with you in this way.

Thank you to my darling spouse, Khara, who since the very first meme I wrote, encouraged me, believed in me, celebrated with me, brainstormed ideas, listened to my stresses and concerns, performed the mundane and yet vitally important house tasks when I was knee-deep in writing deadlines, reminded me of my Higher Self when I didn't have the capacity, and let me cry in their arms when I just needed to let it out. I love you and the life we are building together.

Many thanks to my agent, Meg Thompson, whose early enthusiasm for the message I wanted to communicate with this book gave me the extra boost of confidence I needed to keep going.

Thank you to my editors Michael Szczerban, Thea Diklich-Newell, and Emma Brodie for bringing clarity to my writing and helping me prioritize the reader's needs. Special thanks to Thea for being such a great teammate in the nitty-gritty of nuanced conversation. Additional special thanks to Abimael Ayala-Oquendo for putting so much care into helping me make this book more inclusive, and Ruby Warrington for your much-needed coaching.

Thanks also to other members of the Little, Brown/Voracious team: art director Kirin Diemont, designer Bart Dawson, production editor Pat Jalbert-Levine, and copyeditor Alison Kerr Miller.

I would like to give a heartfelt appreciation to friends who are doing healing work on social media with whom I feel in community. You most likely don't fully know how vital your work is to me on the daily. I see you and appreciate you: James McCrae, Diego Perez, Margeaux Feldman, Jennifer Mulan, adrienne maree brown, Leslie Priscilla, Sah Di Simone, Chani Nicholas, Alexandra Roxo, Kim Saira, Hope Carpenter, and Ruby Warrington.

Thank you to my supporters on social media and the listeners of my podcast. Without your generous spirit and words of encouragement, I could not be doing this. You are so vital.

Thank you to the spiritual guides, healers, and artists who provided a space of belonging when I needed it most.

Thank you to my ancestors, who remind me of my strength, resilience, and sacred connection to Nature.

Thank you to plant medicines, especially Grandmother Ayahuasca for the honor of receiving your wisdom.

And finally, thank you to God for bringing me home every time I stray from Love.

Further Reading

Along my own journey of discovery and healing, and while developing the ideas in *Hello, Higher Self,* I learned from many books and other sources. Here are some texts that I relied on for key facts and historical information, and which may be useful to you as you continue on your own path to understanding and addressing LHBs.

Chapter 1: Social Media
Negative posts get more engagement on social media:

> "Five Points for Anger, One for a 'Like': How Facebook's Formula Fostered Rage and Misinformation" by Jeremy B. Merrill and Will Oremus, *Washington Post*, 2021, https://www.washingtonpost.com /technology/2021/10/26/facebook-angry-emoji-algorithm.

On cancel culture:

> *We Will Not Cancel Us: And Other Dreams of Transformative Justice* by adrienne maree brown (AK Press, 2020).

Chapter 2: Creativity
Historical references to Picasso and appropriation:

> "Picasso, Primitivism, and Cultural Appropriation" by Christopher P. Jones, *Medium,* 2018, https://christopherpjones.medium.com /picasso-primitivism-and-the-rights-and-wrongs-of-cultural -appropriation-1f964fa61cee.

Statistic comparing the sales of art at auctions by gender:

> "Why Is Work by Female Artists Still Valued Less Than Work by Male Artists?" by Taylor Whitten Brown, *Artsy,* 2019, https://www.artsy.net /article/artsy-editorial-work-female-artists-valued-work-male-artists.

Additional reading on accessing your creative voice:

> *The Art of You: The Essential Guidebook for Reclaiming Your Creativity* by James McCrae (Soundstrue, 2023).
> *Bird by Bird* by Anne Lamott (Knopf Doubleday), 2007.

Additional reading on racism in art history:

> *Race and Racism in Nineteenth-Century Art* by Naurice Frank Woods Jr. (University Press of Mississippi, 2021).
>
> *Fearing the Black Body: The Racial Origins of Fat Phobia* by Sabrina Strings (New York University Press, 2021).

Chapter 3: Work and Productivity

Rethinking "laziness":

> *Laziness Does Not Exist* by Devon Price (Atria, 2021).

The effects of stress on child development:

> *The Myth of Normal* by Gabor Maté (Random House UK, 2023).

Cover story featuring Kylie Jenner:

> "At Twenty-One, Kylie Jenner Becomes the Youngest Self-Made Billionaire Ever" by Natalie Robehmed, *Forbes,* 2019, https://www.forbes.com/sites/natalierobehmed/2019/03/05/at-21-kylie-jenner-becomes-the-youngest-self-made-billionaire-ever/?sh=5cc4eb7c2794.

Article claiming Jenner camp embellished earnings:

> "Kylie Jenner's Web of Lies — and Why She's No Longer a Billionaire" by Chase Peterson-Withorn and Madeline Berg, *Forbes,* 2020, https://www.forbes.com/sites/chasewithorn/2020/05/29/inside-kylie-jennerss-web-of-lies-and-why-shes-no-longer-a-billionaire/?sh=f30e57325f7b.

Quote from Gary Vaynerchuk:

> "I Fucking Hate Friday" by Gary Vaynerchuk, 2017, https://garyvaynerchuk.com/fucking-hate-friday.

Quote from Elon Musk:

> Elon Musk on Twitter (X), Nov. 26, 2018, https://twitter.com/elonmusk/status/1067173497909141504?lang=en.

Quote from author David Heinemeier Hansson:

> "Why Are Young People Pretending to Love Work?" by Erin Griffith, *New York Times,* 2019, https://www.nytimes.com/2019/01/26/business/against-hustle-culture-rise-and-grind-tgim.html.

Statistic on workplace discrimination of LGBTQ+ individuals:

> "LGBT People's Experiences of Workplace Discrimination and Harassment," Williams Institute, 2021, https://williamsinstitute.law.ucla.edu/publications/lgbt-workplace-discrimination.

Statistic on lack of employment opportunity for trans folks:

"Protecting and Advancing Health Care for Transgender Adult Communities" by Caroline Medina and Lindsay Mahowald, Center for American Progress, 2021, https://www.americanprogress.org/article /protecting-advancing-health-care-transgender-adult-communities.

Statistic on earning disparities of Black and Latinx versus white workers:

"Earning Disparities by Race and Ethnicity," U.S. Department of Labor, https://www.dol.gov/agencies/ofccp/about/data/earnings /race-and-ethnicity.

Millennial versus baby boomer cost of living:

"Financial Health of Young America: Measuring Generational Declines Between Baby Boomers and Millennials" by Tom Allison, Young Invincibles, 2017, https://younginvincibles.org/wp-content /uploads/2017/04/FHYA-Final2017-1-1.pdf.

Rising healthcare costs statistic:

"Here's How Much the Average American Spends on Health Care" by Ester Bloom, CNBC, 2017, https://www.cnbc.com/2017/06/23 /heres-how-much-the-average-american-spends-on-health-care.html.

Reported success of four-day work week:

"UK Companies in Four-Day Week Pilot Reach Landmark Halfway Point" by Charlotte Lockhart, press release for 4-Day Week Global, 2021, https://www.4dayweek.com/news-posts/uk-four-day-week -pilot-mid-results.

Additional reading on the importance of rest and rethinking productivity:

Rest Is Resistance: A Manifesto by Tricia Hersey (Little, Brown, 2022).

Chapter 4: Money and Abundance

Additional reading on steps to financial literacy and letting go of past narratives around money:

I Will Teach You to Be Rich, 2nd ed., by Ramit Sethi (Workman, 2022).
The Law of Divine Compensation: On Work, Money, and Miracles by Marianne Williamson (HarperCollins, 2014).

Chapter 5: Family and Childhood

References to Samoan culture:

"Samoan Culture: Core Concepts" by Chara Scroope, Cultural Atlas, 2017, https://culturalatlas.sbs.com.au/samoan-culture/samoan-culture-core-concepts.

Additional reading on childhood trauma and family relationships:

The Myth of Normal: Trauma, Illness, and Healing in a Toxic Culture by Gabor Maté (Avery, 2023).

Set Boundaries and Find Peace: A Guide to Reclaiming Yourself by Nedra Glover Tawwab (Penguin, 2021).

Social media accounts addressing trauma that I've found helpful:

Danica Harris, Ph.D., SEP @theempoweredtherapist

Nedra Glover Tawwab, licensed therapist @nedratawwab

Hope Carpenter, @hopehealingarts (feel-good memes)

Margeaux Feldman, @softcore_trauma (more feel-good memes)

Chapter 6: Dating

Research study on ghosting:

"Ghosting and Destiny: Implicit Theories of Relationships Predict Beliefs About Ghosting" by Gili Freedman, Darcey N. Powell, Benjamin Le, and Kipling D. Williams, *Journal of Social and Personal Relationships*, 2018, https://www.researchgate.net/publication/322442819_Ghosting_and_destiny_Implicit_theories_of_relationships_predict_beliefs_about_ghosting.

Dating apps aren't as they seem:

"The Curious Ways Dating Apps Make It Harder to Find Love" by Madeleine A. Fugère, *Psychology Today*, 2019, https://www.psychologytoday.com/us/blog/dating-and-mating/201911/the-curious-ways-dating-apps-make-it-harder-find-love.

Chapter 7: Committed Relationships

Historical background on marriage:

Marriage, a History: How Love Conquered Marriage by Stephanie Coontz, (Penguin, 2006).

Statistic on wives as the primary breadwinner in U.S. households:

"In a Growing Share of U.S. Marriages, Husbands and Wives Earn About the Same" by Richard Fry, Caroline Aragao, Kiley Hurst, and Kim Parker, Pew Research Center, 2023, https://www.pewresearch .org/social-trends/2023/04/13/in-a-growing-share-of-u-s-marriages -husbands-and-wives-earn-about-the-same.

John Bowlby on attachment theory:

A Secure Base: Parent-Child Attachment and Healthy Human Development by John Bowlby (Basic Books, 1988).

Divorce statistic:

"Leading Causes of Divorce: 43 Percent Report Lack of Family Support," by Christy Bieber, *Forbes*, 2023, https://www.forbes.com /advisor/legal/divorce/common-causes-divorce.

Polyamory definition and application to attachment theory:

Polysecure by Jessica Fern (Thorntree, 2020).

Esther Perel on relationships:

Mating in Captivity: Unlocking Erotic Intelligence by Esther Perel (Harper-Collins, 2007).

Chapter 8: Breakups and Being Single

Effects of romantic love on the brain:

"Reward, Addiction, and Emotion Regulation Systems Associated with Rejection in Love" by Helen E. Fisher, Lucy L. Brown, Arthur Aron, Greg Strong, and Debra Mashek, *Journal of Neurophysiology,* 2009, https://journals.physiology.org/doi/full/10.1152/jn.00784.2009.

Katherine Woodward Thomas on breakups:

Conscious Uncoupling: Five Steps to Living Happily Even After by Katherine Woodward Thomas (Harmony, 2016).

Social and legal privileges of married people over single individuals:

"Unearned Privilege: 1,000+ Laws Benefit Only Married People," *Psychology Today,* 2018, https://www.psychologytoday.com/us/blog /living-single/201804/unearned-privilege-1000-laws-benefit-only -married-people.

Unmarried population statistic:

"Unmarried and Single Americans Week: September 17–23," United States Census Bureau, 2023, https://www.census.gov/newsroom

/stories/unmarried-single-americans-week.html#:~:text=From
%20nationalsinglesday.us%2C%20%E2%80%9CDid,those%20who
%20have%20never%20married.

Chapter 9: Friendship

Bias on platonic relationships in scientific research:

> *Friendship: The Evolution, Biology, and Extraordinary Power of Life's Fundamental Bond* by Lydia Denworth (Bloomsbury, 2020).

Additional reading on letting go of cultural myths around friendship:

> *Platonic: How the Science of Attachment Can Help You Make and Keep Friends* by Marisa G. Franco (Penguin, 2022).

Chapter 10: Race and Healing

Historical reference to racial classification:

> "Francios Bernier and the Invention of Racial Classification" by Siep Stuurman, *History Workshop Journal* 50 (2000): 1–21.

Physiological harm due to the stress of racial trauma:

> *The Myth of Normal: Trauma, Illness, and Healing in a Toxic Culture* by Gabor Maté (Penguin, 2023).

Additional reading on racial healing (aimed at therapists and healers):

> *Decolonizing Therapy: Oppression, Historical Trauma, and Politicizing Your Practice* by Dr. Jennifer Mula (W. W. Norton, 2023).
>
> *Do Better: Spiritual Activism for Fighting and Healing from White Supremacy* by Rachel Ricketts (Atria, 2022).

Additional reading on historical racial oppression:

> *The Invention of Humanity: Equality and Cultural Difference in World History* by Siep Stuurman (Harvard University Press, 2017).
>
> *Fearing the Black Body: The Racial Origins of Fat Phobia* by Sabrina Strings (New York University Press, 2021).

Chapter 11: Politics and Activism

Study on trauma survivors and the risk of re-traumatization by media stories:

"Overwhelmed by the News: A Longitudinal Study of Prior
Trauma, Posttraumatic Stress Disorder Trajectories, and News Watch-
ing During the COVID-19 Pandemic" by Zahava Solomon, Karni
Ginzburg, Avi Ohry, and Mario Mikulincer, National Library
of Medicine, 2020, https://www.ncbi.nlm.nih.gov/pmc/articles
/PMC9757611.

Additional reading on compassion, healing, and activism:

All About Love: New Visions by bell hooks (HarperCollins, 2018).
*Do Better: Spiritual Activism for Fighting and Healing from White
Supremacy* by Rachel Ricketts (Atria, 2022).
Pleasure Activism: The Politics of Feeling Good by adrienne maree brown
(AK Press, 2019).

Chapter 12: Beauty and Body Image

Historical references racializing fatness and pathologizing body
hair:

Fearing the Black Body: The Racial Origins of Fat Phobia by Sabrina
Strings (New York University Press, 2019).
Plucked: A History of Hair Removal by Rebecca M. Herzig (New York
University Press, 2016).

History of eugenics movement:

"Eugenics and the Classical Ideal of Beauty in Philip K. Dick's 'The
Golden Man'" by Anne Maxwell, *Science Fiction Studies Journal* 36, no. 1
(2009): 87–100.

Eugenics sterilization statistic:

"The Complicated History of Eugenics in the United States" by Tara
Kibler, *HeinOnline,* 2021, https://home.heinonline.org/blog/2021/06
/the-complicated-history-of-eugenics-in-the-united-states.

Diet culture:

*Anti-Diet: Reclaim Your Time, Money, Well-Being, and Happiness Through
Intuitive Eating* by Christy Harrison (Little, Brown, 2019).

Disordered eating:

"Eating Disorder Statistics," National Association for Anorexia
Nervosa and Associated Disorders, https://anad.org/eating-disorders
-statistics.

Beauty industry:

> "The Ultimate List of Beauty Industry Stats," by Josh Howarth, Explodingtopics.com, 2023, https://explodingtopics.com/blog/beauty-industry-stats.

Body-positive/anti-diet social media accounts I've found helpful:

> Sonalee Rashatwar @fatsextherapist
>
> Ashlee Bennett @bodyimage_therapist

Chapter 13: Sex and Pleasure

Erotic empowerment:

> "Uses of the Erotic: The Erotic as Power," in *Sister Outsider: Essays and Speeches* by Audre Lorde (Crossing, 1984).

On nurturing relationship to genitals:

> *Come As You Are: The Surprising New Science That Will Transform Your Sex Life,* revised and updated, by Emily Nagoski (Simon & Schuster, 2021).

Additional reading on cultural suppression of sexuality:

> *Sex and Punishment: Four Thousand Years of Judging Desire* by Eric Berkowitz (Counterpoint, 2012).

Sexual assault hotlines:

> 800-656-HOPE Rainn.org (U.S.)
>
> 604-245-2425 wavaw.ca (Canada)

Chapter 14: Queerness and the Gender Spectrum

Expansive roles of gender in non-Western cultures:

> "Six Cultures That Recognize More Than Two Genders," *Britannica,* 2023, https://www.britannica.com/list/6-cultures-that-recognize-more-than-two-genders.
>
> "Intersex Definitions," InterACT: Advocates for Intersex Youth, 2021, https://interactadvocates.org/intersex-definitions.

Deconstructing the social construct of gender and sex assignments at birth:

> *Sexing the Body: Gender Politics and the Construction of Sexuality* by Anne Fausto-Sterling (Basic Books, 2000).
>
> *Gender Trouble: Feminism and the Subversion of Identity* by Judith Butler (Routledge, 1990).

Intersex and cultural misconceptions:

> "It's Intersex Awareness Day—Here Are Five Myths We Need to Shatter," Amnesty International, 2018, https://www.amnesty.org/en/latest/news/2018/10/its-intersex-awareness-day-here-are-5-myths-we-need-to-shatter.

Queer discrimination:

> *A Queer History of the United States* by Michael Bronski (Beacon, 2011).
> *Black on Both Sides: A Racial History of Trans Identity* by C. Riley Snorton (University of Minnesota Press, 2017).
> *Sex and Punishment: Four Thousand Years of Judging Desire* by Eric Berkowitz (Counterpoint, 2012).

Chapter 15: Mental Health

Historical diagnosis and treatment of mental illness:

> *Madness in Civilization: A Cultural History of Insanity from the Bible to Freud, from the Madhouse to Modern Medicine* by Andrew Scull (Princeton University Press, 2015).
> "Declared Insane for Speaking Up: The Dark American History of Silencing Women Through Psychiatry" by Kate Moore, *Time,* 2021, https://time.com/6074783/psychiatry-history-women-mental-health.

Mental health stigma:

> "The Stigma of Mental Health and Violence," Disability Rights California, https://www.disabilityrightsca.org/legislation/principles-the-stigma-of-mental-health-and-violence.

Additional reading on how culture affects mental health and mental health treatment:

> *The Myth of Normal: Trauma, Illness, and Healing in a Toxic Culture* by Gabor Maté (Penguin, 2023).
> *Decolonizing Therapy: Oppression, Historical Trauma, and Politicizing Your Practice* by Jennifer Mulan (W.W. Norton, 2023) (aimed at therapists and healers).
> Suicide & Crisis Lifeline (U.S. and Canada): Call or text 988.

Chapter 16: Spirituality

Appropriation in Western spiritual and wellness circles:

Who Is Wellness For?: An Examination of Wellness Culture and Who It Leaves Behind by Fariha Roisin (HarperCollins, 2022).

Ram Dass anecdote:

Being Ram Dass by Ram Dass (Sounds True, 2022).

Additional reading on spirituality and healing:

Lighter: Let Go of the Past, Connect with the Present, Expand the Future by yung pueblo (Harmony Books, 2022).

A New Earth: Awakening to Your Life's Purpose by Eckhart Tolle (Penguin, 2005).

Radical Acceptance: Embracing Your Life with the Heart of a Buddha by Tara Brach (Random House, 2004).

You Were Born for This: Astrology for Radical Self-Acceptance by Chani Nicholas (HarperCollins, 2020).

About the Author

Bunny Michael is a multidisciplinary queer Mexican/Samoan artist and influencer who has inspired an audience of more than 250,000 Instagram followers to discover their Higher Self. They are the host of the XO Higher Self podcast, and their work has also been featured in the *New York Times, Huffpo, Paper Magazine, Dazed & Confused,* and *ID.* They currently reside in upstate New York with their spouse, Khara, and pets Rio and Zoro.